Foot Orthotics
in
Therapy and Sport

Skip Hunter, PT, ATC
Clemson Sports Medicine and Rehabilitation Clinic

Michael G. Dolan, MA, ATC, CSCS
Canisius College, Buffalo, New York

John M. Davis, PT, ATC
University of North Carolina at Chapel Hill

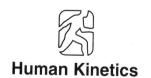

Human Kinetics

Library of Congress Cataloging-in-Publication Data

Hunter, Skip, 1948-
   Foot orthotics in therapy and sport / Skip Hunter, Michael G.
Dolan, John M. Davis.
    p. cm.
   Includes bibliographical references and index.
   ISBN 87322-829-4 (pbk.)
   1. Orthopedic shoes. 2. Foot--Abnormalities. 3. Sports medicine.
I. Dolan, Michael G., 1959- . II. Davis, John M., 1951-
III. Title.
   [DNLM: 1. Orthotic Devices. 2. Foot Deformities--therapy.
3. Foot Injuries--therapy. 4. Biomechanics. 5. Equipment Design.
WE 26 H947f 1995]
RD757.S45H86 1995
617.3'98--dc20
DNLM/DLC
for Library of Congress   95-2243
                              CIP

ISBN: 0-87322-829-4

Notice: As new scientific information becomes available through basic and clinical research, recommended treatments and therapies undergo changes. The authors and publisher have done everything possible to make this book accurate, up-to-date, and in accord with accepted standards at the time of publication. Any application of the recommendations set forth in the following pages is at the reader's discretion and sole risk.

Acquisitions Editor: Rick Frey, PhD; **Developmental Editor:** Christine Drews; **Assistant Editors:** Karen Bojda, Rebecca Ewert, and John Wentworth; **Editorial Assistant:** Karen Grieves; **Copyeditor:** Karl Stull; **Proofreader:** Dena Popara; **Indexer:** Kathy Bennett; **Typesetter:** Francine Hamerski; **Text Designer:** Judy Henderson; **Layout Artists:** Francine Hamerski and Robert Reuther; **Photo Editor:** Boyd LaFoon; **Cover Designer:** Jack Davis; **Photographer (interior):** Jessica Miller; **Illustrator:** Nicolé A. Barbuto; **Printer:** United Graphics

Printed in the United States of America   10 9 8 7 6 5 4 3 2 1

Human Kinetics
P.O. Box 5076, Champaign, IL 61825-5076
1-800-747-4457

Canada: Human Kinetics, Box 24040, Windsor, ON N8Y 4Y9
1-800-465-7301 (in Canada only)

Europe: Human Kinetics, P.O. Box IW14, Leeds LS16 6TR, England
(44) 532 781708

Australia: Human Kinetics, 2 Ingrid Street, Clapham 5062, South Australia
(08) 371 3755

New Zealand: Human Kinetics, P.O. Box 105-231, Auckland 1
(09) 309 2259

I dedicate this book to the memory of Dr. Joseph DeWalt.
His faith in me allowed my career to prosper.

SH

To my Mom and Dad for always leading by example
and to Kristen for her love and support.

MGD

Dedicated to the memory of Dr. Joe DeWalt,
an unsung pioneer in sports medicine.

JMD

Contents

Foreword

A number of years ago, I had the pleasure of working with a team physician who repeatedly and emphatically stressed the idea that the cause of many of the injuries seen in the lower extremity can be traced directly to some structural deformity or biomechanical abnormality of the foot. Through my experiences in dealing with athletes, as an athletic trainer and physical therapist, I have come to realize the accuracy of this approach in evaluation and management of many of the injuries that occur in the lower extremity.

The authors of this text—one a colleague, one a former colleague, and one a former graduate student—are all practicing clinicians who over the years have demonstrated a genuine interest and considerable expertise in designing and constructing orthotic devices for their patients. As with many of the techniques we all routinely practice in sports medicine, orthoses reflects some combination of both art and science. In this text, the authors have focused their emphasis on the art of making orthotics.

The sports medicine and podiatric communities have recommended various types of orthotics. This text is a compilation of the most current theories, approaches, and techniques for manufacturing orthotics. It will serve as a practical guide for the clinician interested in gaining additional knowledge and expertise in choosing an appropriate orthotic for individual patients. This text fills a void in the sports medicine literature, and I commend the authors for their effort.

William E. Prentice, PhD, PT, ATC

Preface

Our purpose in writing this book was to raise the interest of those clinicians who are not currently working with orthotics or who may be using different techniques. When I first moved to the University of North Carolina in 1979, the athletic training staff decided that each of the staff PT/ATCs would specialize in a particular area. Since I was the new person on the staff, I was assigned feet. I started by taking an excellent course by Michael Wooden in Atlanta. Then I made my first pair of orthotics in the household toaster oven. The second pair I ever made, I set on fire in the household toaster oven. But I learned something every time I made an orthotic, and I got progressively better. As I tell all my patients, making an orthotic is an art, not a science. Once all the measurements are taken, the artistic side of things starts.

Had my kindergarten teacher not had pity on me, I would not have passed drawing and cutting. So how do I make orthotics now? Just as with anything else in the sports world—practice and repetition. You would not want to have worn any of the first 50 or so orthotics I made. But I kept trying, and now, after a few thousand, I think I am pretty good. The point is this: Don't be afraid to try.

The jargon used in foot and ankle science can be pretty scary. We have tried to write this book in such a way that the starting practitioner and the practitioner who has only dabbled in orthotics will find something useful. Please keep in mind: We are not podiatrists or physicians. Some foot problems are complex and need to be seen higher up the chain of clinical practice. Many of the orthotics described here are temporary in nature. These may be used to ascertain the need for longer-lasting orthotics. Neither is this book meant to be a deep biomechanical discussion. There are many excellent books on the market for this purpose, and we recommend that serious readers who find this book interesting purchase a good biomechanical text. A firm foundation in biomechanics will be of immense value in the understanding of orthotic therapy.

A majority of the orthotics we make are for sports usage, although these orthotics may be adapted for other applications. We hope this text will serve as the sports clinician's introduction to orthotics and that it may carry over into the treatment of other problems as well.

Skip Hunter, PT, ATC

Acknowledgments

When we first started writing this book, we never thought it would be this involved and time-consuming. We would like to thank several people for their contributions to this textbook. Rick Frey of Human Kinetics who, when we approached him, encouraged three clinicians to write a book. Ms. Christine Drews, our developmental editor, took our project in midstride and ran with it. If not for her professional guidance and enthusiastic attitude, this project would still be on the table. We may owe her the biggest thank-you of all.

Two young ladies have contributed major portions of this textbook. Ms. Jessica Miller is responsible for the photography in this text. One of our goals in writing this text was to make it easy to see how we make orthotics. Jessica's photographs allowed us to take what we do in the clinic and training room and put it into pictures. Ms. Nicole Barbuto, an aspiring medical illustrator, is responsible for the line art in the text. She has taken complex anatomical and biomechanical concepts and made them easy to see and understand.

Special thanks to Robert Duggan, DPM, ATC and Robert Moore, PhD, PT, ATC who provided critical review and insight as they reviewed the text. Their professional criticism and input has added to the quality of the text.

Lastly, we would like to acknowledge a group of colleagues—doctors, physical therapists, athletic trainers, podiatrists, and students—who have added to this text by influencing our clinical practice, especially in the areas of foot examination and fabrication of foot orthotics: Dr. Joe DeWalt, Dr. Phillip Bach, Dr. Bob Duggan, Dr. Stephen Joyce, Dr. Bernie Rohrbacher, Dr. Larry Bowman, Jim Blanton, Heather Janine Iman, Pete Koehneke, Bill Prentice, Amy Schule, Paul Spear, Phil Tonsoline, and Lori Whitlow.

Introduction to Orthotic Therapy

The use of foot orthotic devices in physical therapy and sports medicine settings has increased dramatically as a means of treating pathology of the lower kinetic chain. To understand why, let's begin with the basics, as this chapter introduces and overviews the terminology, function, indications, and types of foot orthotic devices and relates these issues to the contemporary use of orthotic devices in a clinical setting.

Definition of Orthotic Devices

We define a foot orthotic as a device that is placed in a person's shoe to reduce or eliminate pathological stresses to the foot or other portions of the lower kinetic chain. These stresses include structural and positional deformities, lack of shock absorption, and excessive shearing forces. However, ours is by no means the last word in definitions. With health care professionals from a variety of disciplines now actively involved in the fabrication of orthotic devices, there is some confusion in regard to nomenclature. Notably, there is no single accepted definition of the term orthotic as it relates to clinical practice. *Stedman's Medical Dictionary* defines orthosis as the correction of maladjustments. It defines orthotics as the science that deals with the making and fitting of orthopedic appliances. Carter (1987) defines an orthotic as a device that applies force to a body segment to correct a mobile deformity and to stabilize, protect, or motorize (permit motion in) a joint or body area. The literature abounds with other definitions, each with its own special nomenclature.

- Jahss (1991) states that an orthotic is "a mechanical device made for the foot or toes that is used to either stabilize the foot or hold it in an optimal position, increase function, limit motion of a painful joint, decrease weight bearing on painful areas, or protect the foot or toes from pressure or excess friction against each other or the shoe."

- D'Ambrosia (1985) defines an orthotic as a device that aligns an improperly balanced foot by controlling subtalar motion.

- James, Bates, and Osternig (1978) define an orthotic as a "shim" placed between the foot and shoe to position the foot near its neutral subtalar joint position so it can function more efficiently.

- Donatelli and Wooden (1990) posit that the function of a biomechanical orthotic is to control excessive and potentially harmful subtalar and midtarsal joint movement.

- Smith, Clarke, Hamill, and Santopietro (1986), on the other hand, conducted research with different types of orthotics and concluded that the devices affect the velocity and amount of calcaneal eversion as a component of pronation.

At this point, variation among individual practitioners and patients' circumstances is to be expected. Moreover, there may be singular or multiple indications for prescription of foot orthotic devices. We encourage our readers to formulate their own *working* definition that is consistent with their clinical practice.

It is critical to realize that orthotic devices are not a panacea for lower extremity injuries and must not be considered a treatment for all pathologies of the lower kinetic chain. Rather, orthotic devices should be used when a structural or a positional foot deformity, lack of shock absorption, or excessive shear force is (1) documented by clinical examination and (2) contributes to pathology. Once the clinical decision is made to include an orthotic device in the management of the condition, the orthotic must be regarded as one part of the entire treatment plan. The importance of a comprehensive approach, including appropriate medical intervention, therapeutic exercise, therapeutic modalities, and modifications of activities, cannot be overemphasized in a successful rehabilitation and reconditioning program. For all the benefit that appropriate use of an orthotic device can have in reducing or eliminating symptoms, inappropriate use of foot orthotics when not indicated or incorrectly fitted can cause an increase of symptoms, abnormal stresses on other parts of the lower kinetic chain, and in some cases, frank injury.

Indications for Use of Orthotic Devices

Foot orthotic devices are indicated in a variety of orthopedic injuries commonly encountered in physical therapy and athletic training. The indications for foot orthotics include but are not limited to structural and positional imbalances of the foot, lack of shock absorption, pressure-sensitive areas, shearing forces, and unique orthopedic and sport injuries. The decision to use an orthotic device must be based on a complete history, biomechanical examination, and the individual needs of the patient or athlete.

Structural and Positional Imbalances of the Foot Contributing to Lower Kinetic Chain Injuries

The foot is an adaptable unit that can accommodate changes in terrain surface as well as become a firm lever for push-off. Structural and positional deformities of the foot or lower kinetic chain in-

fluence the function of the foot during its gait cycle. Examples of structural deformities include forefoot varus, forefoot valgus, rearfoot varus, rearfoot valgus, tibial varum, and so on. These deformities are not in themselves pathological to the lower kinetic chain, unless the foot compensates for these deformities in an abnormal or excessive fashion. Root, Orien, and Weed (1977) categorize compensation by the foot as either normal or abnormal. Normal compensation is an adjustment to changes in the surface of terrain. Abnormal compensation occurs when the foot adjusts for abnormal structure or function of the trunk or lower extremity. In addition, depending on the degree and type of deformity, the degree of compensatory motion is classified as fully compensated, partially compensated, or uncompensated. Foot orthotics are indicated to decrease abnormal compensation. The most frequent compensatory movement resulting from structural or positional deformities is subtalar joint pronation. Pronation is represented by plantar flexion and adduction of the talus and eversion of the calcaneus in a closed kinetic chain position. One study of subjects classified as pronators who wore orthotic devices found that the orthotic devices decreased the period of pronation and amount of maximal pronation (Bates, Osternig, Mason, & James, 1979). Retrospective studies (Donatelli, Hurlbert, Conaway, & St. Pierre, 1988; Gross, Davlin, & Evanski, 1991) have shown that orthotic devices are effective in returning most individuals to previous levels of activity.

Shock Absorption

One of the primary functions of an orthotic device is to provide shock absorption during walking, running, or athletic activity. Running applies force equivalent to two to three times a person's body weight (Mann, 1985).

Lack of shock absorption is frequently seen in athletes with a cavus foot and exhibiting abnormal supination. The associated lack of normal subtalar joint pronation deprives the lower kinetic chain of the terrain adaptability and shock absorption value of this movement. These athletes are difficult to treat and most frequently are fitted with a soft orthotic to increase shock absorption and cushioning (see Figure 1.1).

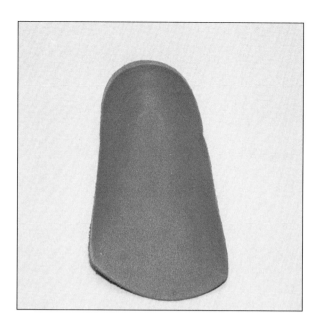

Figure 1.1 A soft orthotic to increase shock absorption.

Therapeutic shock absorption can be achieved using various materials, as is reflected in research. Brodsky, Kourosh, Stills, and Mooney (1988) tested five materials commonly used for shoe inserts and found that all were effective in reducing force over a simulated bony prominence. Campbell, Newell, and McLure (1982), testing 31 shoe-insert materials for compression and deformation characteristics, concluded that moderately deformable materials are best suited for clinical usage. McPoil and Cornwall (1992) examined plantar pressures with subjects wearing insoles constructed of three common types of materials: PPT, Spenco, and Viscolas. Forefoot plantar pressures were reduced with all three materials and rearfoot pressures were reduced with the Spenco and PPT. Jørgensen (1990) found that a well-fitting stiff heel counter significantly reduced muscle load on heel strike during running. These are excellent examples of how simple, commercially available appliances are effective in reducing and managing pain in common orthopedic conditions that are frequently encountered in physical therapy or an athletic training setting.

Pressure-Sensitive Areas

Simple orthotic devices can be fabricated to relieve pressure-sensitive areas of the foot. The use of orthopedic felt or foam is an easy, inexpensive, and efficient method of reducing pressure to areas of the foot. Various forms of orthotics that transfer weightbearing stresses to painless areas are frequently used (Wu, 1990). In addition, a soft orthotic may be fabricated with a relief area cut out to reduce pressure on the plantar aspect of the foot (Figure 1.2). Using material such as Plastazote under areas of the foot that are bearing excessive weight can redistribute stresses during gait (Schwartz, 1990).

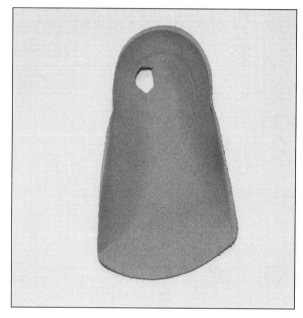

Figure 1.2 Soft orthotic with cutout to reduce pressure on painful area of calcaneus.

Shearing Forces

Abnormal or excessive shearing forces can contribute to common conditions of the foot such as blisters, calluses, corns, and more debilitating conditions such as interdigital neuromas. Shearing calluses are associated with abnormal distribution of forces among the hallux and lesser metatarsals (Root et al., 1977). The use of materials such as Spenco or PPT is a quick and efficient method of reducing shearing forces to the foot that contribute to calluses, blisters, and abnormal contact between the foot and shoe. In addition, orthotics that improve the biomechanical function of the foot and thereby restore normal motion will decrease adverse shearing forces to the foot.

Special Orthopedic and Athletic Conditions

Special foot orthotics can be constructed and used as an integral part of the treatment of a variety of orthopedic injuries to the foot and lower kinetic chain that affect athletes and nonathletes alike. Combs-Orteza, Vogelbach, and Denegar (1992) used molded orthotics on patients with acute ankle sprains and found a reduction in pain during jogging. They speculated that maintaining the foot in a more neutral position produced less strain on the lateral ligaments which may result in improved kinesthetic/proprioceptive feedback. Chapter 9 discusses how orthotic devices can be used in the management of such conditions as rheumatoid arthritis, turf toe, metatarsalgia, plantar fasciitis, and interdigital neuromas.

Parts of an Orthotic

Philips (1990) has broken the functional orthotic into four specific units: the shell, post, forefoot extension, and cover.

Shell

The shell of an orthotic is the primary material or materials from which the device is fabricated. The rigidity of the material determines whether the orthotic device is classified as rigid, semirigid, or soft (see Figure 1.3). The selection of the shell material must be based on the individual needs of the patient or athlete. These considerations include the amount of biomechanical control needed, athletic or functional demands, body weight, and type of shoes.

Post

The post is the portion of the orthotic that is used to control abnormal movement. Orthotic devices usually comprise a forefoot and rearfoot post (see Figure 1.4). The rearfoot post is used to control movement of the calcaneus at heel strike (Donatelli & Wooden, 1990) (see Figure 1.5). The forefoot post is used to support the forefoot and decrease the need for compensatory and abnormal subtalar and midtarsal joint movements. The term "bringing the floor up to the foot" helps explain the concept of forefoot posting. Figure 1.6a illustrates the common deformity of forefoot varus and the accompanying compensatory pronation that can result. The function of the posted orthotic, in this case a varus post, is to bring the floor up to the medial portion of the foot so that the subtalar joint will not have to pronate beyond neutral, thus allowing the foot to function in a more biomechanically correct position (see Figure 1.6b).

A post can either be extrinsic or intrinsic. An extrinsic post is material added to the bottom of the orthotic, usually a wedge-shaped piece of foam or cork, to control abnormal movement. Extrinsic

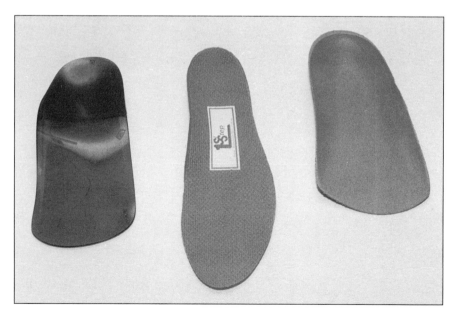

Figure 1.3 Rigid, semirigid, and soft orthotic shells.

posts are most commonly used in the fabrication of semirigid orthotics, as shown in Figure 1.7. Extrinsic posts are easy to modify by adding or grinding down the material. This allows for minor adjustments of the device. In addition, if the post is mispositioned it can be removed and put back onto the orthotic in the proper place with minimal effort and time. The disadvantage to extrinsic posting is that it can make the orthotic rather bulky and difficult to get into a shoe. An intrinsic post is built into the orthotic, typically by modifying a positive mold to correct for biomechanical abnormalities. No material is added to the bottom of the orthotic device (Figure 1.8).

Posts

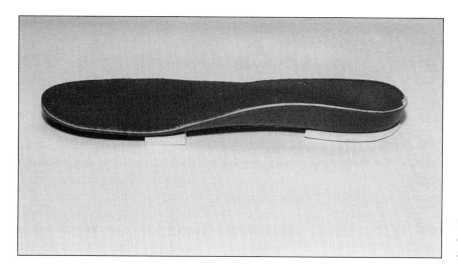

Figure 1.4 Semirigid orthotic with forefoot and rearfoot posts.

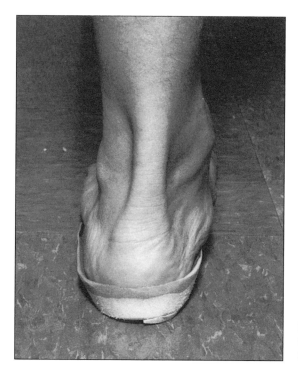

Figure 1.5 Rearfoot post controls the calcaneus at heel strike.

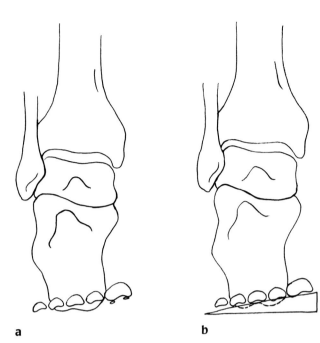

a   b

Figure 1.6   (a) Forefoot varus deformity; (b) Varus post corrects the deformity by "bringing the floor up to the foot."

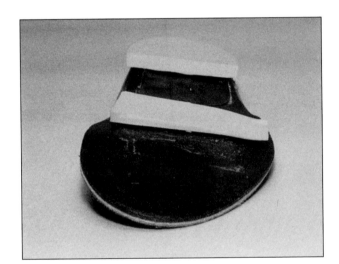

Figure 1.7   Semirigid orthotic with extrinsic posts at the forefoot and rearfoot.

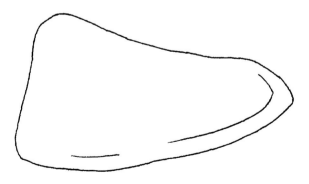

Figure 1.8   Orthotic with intrinsic forefoot post.

The approach of undercorrecting in the fabrication of posts has found support among experienced practitioners who emphasize that posting the forefoot and rearfoot to full measurements is seldom indicated (McKenzie, Clement, & Taunton, 1985). We rarely attempt to correct the entire deformity with the use of a post. We typically undercorrect the deformity to ensure that the orthotic device will fit inside the person's shoe and be comfortable during gait and athletic competition. The use of extrinsically posted semirigid orthotics allows the clinician to increase or decrease the post in response to clinical improvement and patient input. Donatelli et al. (1988), posting forefoot varus to 61 percent and rearfoot deformity to 57 percent of the measured deformity, report excellent clinical results. Recently, Johanson, Donatelli, Wooden, Andrew, and Cummings (1994) compared the effects of posting just the forefoot alone, rearfoot alone, and both combined and found that the combination of a forefoot and rearfoot post was most effective in controlling pronation. Opinions vary regarding the optimal use of posts; this is an area of clinical treatment that requires further study. We usually post both the forefoot and rearfoot when our goal is correction of a structural or positional imbalance.

Forefoot Extension

The majority of the orthotics that we fabricate for use in an athletic population are three-quarter length, running from the calcaneus to the metatarsal heads. Occasionally a forefoot extension is used to cover the entire plantar surface of the foot (see Figure 1.9). Most soft orthotics, as well as many prefabricated devices, whose primary function is shock absorption are full length.

Cover

The cover is applied over the top of the orthotic device (Figure 1.10). The cover serves three primary purposes: making the orthotic device more durable, adding shock absorption properties inherent in some of the materials on the market, and making the orthotic more attractive.

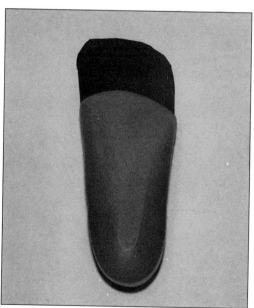

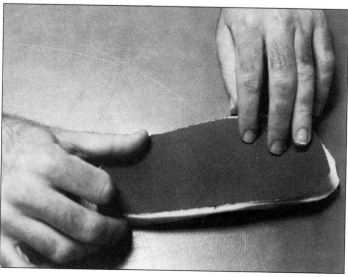

Figure 1.9 A forefoot extension added to a three-quarter length orthotic.

Figure 1.10 Semirigid orthotic device with a cover.

Types of Orthotic Devices

There are various ways to classify foot orthoses. For example, Schwartz (1990) divides foot orthotics according to method of fabrication, reason for manufacture, and materials used in manufacture. Unfortunately, the terms that have been used to describe orthotic devices are varied and sometimes redundant. For the purposes of this book, orthotics are best broken into three distinct groups—rigid, semirigid, and soft—based on the physical properties of the materials used in the fabrication of the shell.

Rigid Orthotics

Rigid orthotics are made of nonflexible acrylics or graphite materials such as TL-61 or Plexidure. Rigid orthotics are prescribed when absolute biomechanical control of structural deformities is indicated. In a clinical setting, fabrication of rigid orthotics is the most difficult of the three types due to the unforgiving nature of the material. In fabricating a rigid orthotic, the neutral position of the subtalar joint is captured via a negative cast, from which a positive mold is created. The positive molds are then modified to correct for biomechanical or positional abnormalities. This allows for intrinsic posting of the device as opposed to extrinsic posting, which is the norm for semirigid and soft orthotics. Modification of a positive mold includes adding or removing plaster to or from the molds. This process is time consuming and requires special training by the clinician. The acrylic or graphite material is then heated and molded over the positive cast. Certain rigid and semirigid materials can be molded directly onto the patient's foot with the subtalar joint held in neutral position, as described by Combs-Orteza et al. (1992). It is critical that the clinician has knowledge of the physical properties of the materials to ensure patient safety and comfort.

We seldom make rigid orthotics in our clinical settings due to the complexity and time consuming nature of the process. When a rigid device is indicated, we send a negative cast of the neutral subtalar joint position with the appropriate orthotic prescription to one of the multitude of orthotic manufacturing laboratories. The rigidity of these appliances can make them unsuitable for athletes who participate in sports that require sprinting or high-speed cutting. However, we have seen athletes who participate in these types of sports (basketball, football, etc.) adapt well to rigid orthotic devices. This reinforces the concept that patients should be treated for their individual needs and not with general treatment assumptions. Rigid orthotics are frequently used in the management of adolescent conditions, though the effectiveness of these devices remains controversial (Mereday, Dolan, & Lusskin, 1972; Penneau, Lutter, & Winter, 1982). Examples of rigid foot orthotics include the University of California Biomechanical Laboratory (UCBL) device, Shaffer plates, heel stabilizers, and the Whitman-Robert orthotic.

Semirigid Orthotics

The majority of orthotics that we fabricate in our clinical settings are classified as semirigid. Semirigid orthotics are made from a wide variety of materials, such as low-temperature thermoplastics, foams, corks, leather, and covering material. Usually extrinsic posts are added to the semirigid orthotic to correct structural foot imbalances, allowing the subtalar and midtarsal joints to function efficiently in the stance portion of gait. However, it is possible to fabricate semirigid devices with an intrinsic forefoot post (Colonna, 1989). This procedure involves modification of the positive mold, as in the manufacture of rigid orthotics.

Among the advantages of semirigid orthotics is that they provide support for controlling abnormal and excessive motion at the subtalar and midtarsal joints while adding shock-absorption properties for the lower kinetic chain. In addition, the materials are easy to work with and modify, allowing for subtle corrections to the forefoot and rearfoot posting as well as to the length and width of the orthotic device. This adaptability is particularly critical to meeting the needs of the athletic population, whose shoe designs and athletic demands vary by sport. Semirigid orthotics can be fabricated with medial and lateral flares that prevent the tendency of the foot to slide off the orthotic (McPoil & Brocato, 1985). Slippage is a common complaint from athletic patients fitted with rigid orthotics. Most runners need a flexible orthosis for faster speeds, according to Subotnick (1975).

Our rationale in fabricating semirigid orthotics is that they should both provide support and control excessive movement while allowing the normal pronation and supination required in activities of daily living and in athletics (such as sprinting and lateral movements). Semirigid orthotics can serve as temporary orthotics, enabling fine adjustments in posting (Donatelli et al., 1988). After a successful trial period, a permanent pair can be fabricated or ordered. However, many temporary orthotics become permanent orthotics because the patient and clinician like the temporary pair and feel concern about increasing symptoms by switching to another device.

Soft Orthotics

The primary purposes of soft orthotics are shock absorption, relief of pressure areas, and relief from shearing forces to the plantar aspect of the foot. Soft orthotics are inexpensive, easy to fabricate, and effective in the management of many types of orthopedic injuries. A wide variety of materials, discussed in chapter 9, is available to the clinician for fabricating soft orthotics. Eng and Pierrynowski (1993) used soft orthotics constructed of Spenco insoles, with rubber wedges used as the post material, on patients with pronated feet and patellofemoral syndrome. Their results suggest that the soft orthotics, in addition to an exercise program, were effective in managing this common orthopedic condition. McPoil (1983) discusses the fabrication of the cobra pad as an inexpensive and effective device manufactured from soft materials such as Spenco or PPT. The cobra pad is used in the management of a forefoot varus or valgus deformity. In the case of a forefoot varus deformity, the thick portion would be located on the medial aspect of the foot in a fashion similar to an extrinsic post added to a semirigid or soft orthotic. The cobra pad can be fabricated in 10 to 15 minutes with the patient able to use the pad immediately. The material is easy to work with and thereby allows easy adjustment of the pad. A major advantage of soft orthotics such as the cobra pad is that the patient can wear the device home immediately after fabrication.

Fabrication of Orthotic Devices

A multitude of fabrication methods is available to clinicians, ranging from simple to complex, inexpensive to costly, and quick to time consuming. Readers must use the system that they believe is most effective and suitable to their clinical skills and practice. Our preference is for semirigid orthotic devices that we fabricate in-house. Other clinicians have had success using other techniques described in this text.

For clinicians who choose to fabricate their own orthotic devices, the following skills and equipment will get you started:

- Evaluation techniques and the ability to assess neutral subtalar joint position
- Experience with the materials to be used in fabrication
- A minimum work area of approximately 150 square feet
- A basic laboratory set-up, which will cost approximately $1,000–1,200
- The willingness to give it a try

Summary

This chapter introduced the basic terminology, indications, and types of orthotic devices used in a clinical setting that will be expanded upon in the following chapters. Rapid advancements in foot biomechanics research, examination methods, and fabrication techniques require clinicians to remain well informed on contemporary trends. Clinicians who incorporate the use of foot orthotics into clinical practice must evaluate a multitude of variables and determine what is most suitable for their setting. Working with individuals who need foot orthotic devices is professionally challenging. Orthotics can be effective in the management of injuries frequently encountered in physical therapy and athletic training settings.

References

Bates, B.T., Osternig, L.R., Mason, B., & James, S.L. (1979). Foot orthotic devices to modify selected aspects of lower extremity mechanics. *The American Journal of Sports Medicine*, **7**(6), 338–342.

Brodsky, J.W., Kourosh, S., Stills, M., & Mooney, V. (1988). Objective evaluation of insert material for diabetic and athletic footwear. *Foot and Ankle*, **9**, 111–116.

Campbell, G., Newell, E., & McLure, M. (1982). Compression testing of foamed plastics and rubbers for use as orthotic shoe insoles. *Prosthetics and Orthotics International*, **6**, 48–52.

Carter, G. (1987). Foot orthoses. *Australian Family Physician*, **16**, 1104–1108.

Colonna, P. (1989). Fabrication of a custom molded orthotic using an intrinsic posting technique for a forefoot varus deformity. *Physical Therapy Forum*, **8**, 6–7.

Combs-Orteza, L., Vogelbach, D.W., & Denegar, C.R. (1992). The effect of molded and unmolded orthotics on balance and pain while jogging following inversion ankle sprain. *The Journal of Athletic Training*, **27**, 80–84.

D'Ambrosia, R.D. (1985). Orthotic devices in running injuries. *Clinics in Sports Medicine*, **4**(4), 611–618.

Donatelli, R., Hurlbert, C., Conaway, D., & St. Pierre, R. (1988). Biomechanical foot orthotics: A retrospective study. *The Journal of Orthopaedic and Sports Physical Therapy*, **10**, 205–212.

Donatelli, R., & Wooden, M. (1990). Biomechanical orthotics. In R. Donatelli (Ed.), *The biomechanics of the foot and ankle* (pp. 193–216). Philadelphia: Davis.

Eng, J.J., & Pierrynowski, M.R. (1993). Evaluation of soft foot orthotics in the treatment of patellofemoral pain syndrome. *Physical Therapy*, **73**(2), 62–70.

Gross, M.L., Davlin, L.B., & Evanski, P.M. (1991). Effectiveness of orthotic shoe inserts in the long-distance runner. *The American Journal of Sports Medicine*, **19**(4), 409–412.

Jahss, M. (1991). Arch supports, shielding, and orthodigita. In M. Jahss (Ed.), *Disorders of the foot and ankle* (pp. 2857–2865). Philadelphia: Sanders.

James, S.L., Bates, B.T., & Osternig, L.R. (1978). Injuries to runners. *The American Journal of Sports Medicine*, **6**, 40–50.

Johanson, M.A., Donatelli, R., Wooden, M.J., Andrew, P.D., & Cummings, G.S. (1994). Effects of three different posting methods on controlling abnormal subtalar pronation. *Physical Therapy*, **74**(2), 149–161.

Jørgensen, U. (1990). Body load in heel-strike running: The effect of a firm heel counter. *The American Journal of Sports Medicine*, **18**, 177–181.

Mann, R.A. (1985). Biomechanics of the foot. In W.H. Bunch et al. (Eds.), *Atlas of orthotics*, 2nd. (pp. 112–125) St. Louis: Mosby.

McKenzie, D.C., Clement, D.B., & Taunton, J.E. (1985). Running shoes, orthotics, and injuries. *Sports Medicine*, **2**, 334–347.

McPoil, T.G. (1983). The cobra pad: An orthotic alternative for the physical therapist. *The Journal of Orthopaedic and Sports Physical Therapy*, **5**, 30–32.

McPoil, T.G., & Brocato, R.S. (1985). The foot and ankle: Biomechanical evaluation and treatment. In J.A. Gould & G.J. Davies (Eds.), *Orthopaedic and sports physical therapy* (Vol. 2, pp. 313–341). St. Louis: Mosby.

McPoil, T.G., & Cornwall, M.W. (1992). Effect of insole material on force and plantar pressures during walking. *Journal of American Podiatric Medical Association*, **82**(8), 412–416.

Mereday, C., Dolan, C.M.E., & Lusskin, R. (1972). Evaluation of the University of California Biomechanics Laboratory shoe insert in "flexible" pes planus. *Clinical Orthopedics and Related Research*, **82**, 45–58.

Penneau, K., Lutter, L.D., & Winter, R.D. (1982). Pes planus: Radiographic changes with foot orthoses and shoes. *Foot & Ankle*, **2**, 299–302.

Philips, J.W. (1990). *The functional foot orthosis*. New York: Churchill Livingstone.

Root, M., Orien, W., & Weed, J. (1977). *Clinical biomechanics: Vol. II. Normal and abnormal function of the foot*. Los Angeles: Clinical Biomechanics.

Schwartz, N. (1990). The diabetic foot. In R. Donatelli (Ed.), *The biomechanics of the foot and ankle* (pp. 178–189). Philadelphia: Davis.

Smith, L.S., Clarke, T.E., Hamill, C.L., & Santopietro, F. (1986). The effects of soft and semi-rigid orthoses upon rearfoot movement in running. *Journal of the American Podiatric Medical Association*, **76**, 227–233.

Subotnick, S. (1975). The abuses of orthotic devices. *The Journal of the American Podiatry Association*, **65**, 1025–1027.

Wu, K.K. (1990). *Foot orthoses: Principles and clinical application*. Baltimore: Williams & Wilkins.

2

Relation of Foot Biomechanics to Lower Extremity Pathology

The foot must function as a jack of all trades. It must be a loose adapter for uneven terrain, while at the same time be a rigid lever to provide push-off. The foot must also absorb some of the rotation of the lower extremity so that rotation can occur in the hips and pelvis, and so that the foot itself does not have to rotate (D'Ambrosia & Douglas, 1982; McPoil & Knecht, 1985). Figure 2.1 shows the bones and joints of the lower kinetic chain; Figure 2.2 focuses on those of the foot.

Conversely, when abnormal foot biomechanics are present, the inability to absorb rotation or be a "torque converter" causes rotation to pass upward in the other direction (Donatelli, 1985; Lundberg, Svensson, Byland, Goldie, & Selvik, 1989).

This chapter reviews the literature on the effects of abnormal foot biomechanics on the lower extremity. It is not meant to be a full treatise on biomechanics but rather an explanation of the mechanisms by which orthotics may affect the lower extremity.

Pronation and Supination

The subtalar joint consists of three articulations between the talus and calcaneus. The terms pronation and supination were first used to describe the motion of the subtalar joint by Manter (1941). Pronation of the foot is a triplane movement that occurs normally at the subtalar joint. In a weight-bearing or closed kinetic chain, the talus adducts and the plantar aspect flexes, while the calcaneus everts on the talus (Figure 2.3). In open chain pronation, the calcaneus moves into dorsiflexion, abduction, and eversion without movement of the talus.

Supination is also a triplane movement that occurs normally at the subtalar joint. In weightbearing stance, this movement is the opposite of pronation. The calcaneus inverts while the talus abducts and dorsiflexes (Figure 2.4). In open chain supination, the calcaneus moves into plantar flexion, adduction, and inversion without movement of the talus (Root, Orien, & Weed, 1977).

This chapter is adapted from Hunter, S. (1991). The relationship of foot biomechanics to knee pain, and the use of orthotics. *Postgraduate Studies in Sports Physical Therapy.* Berryhill, VA: Forum Medicum.

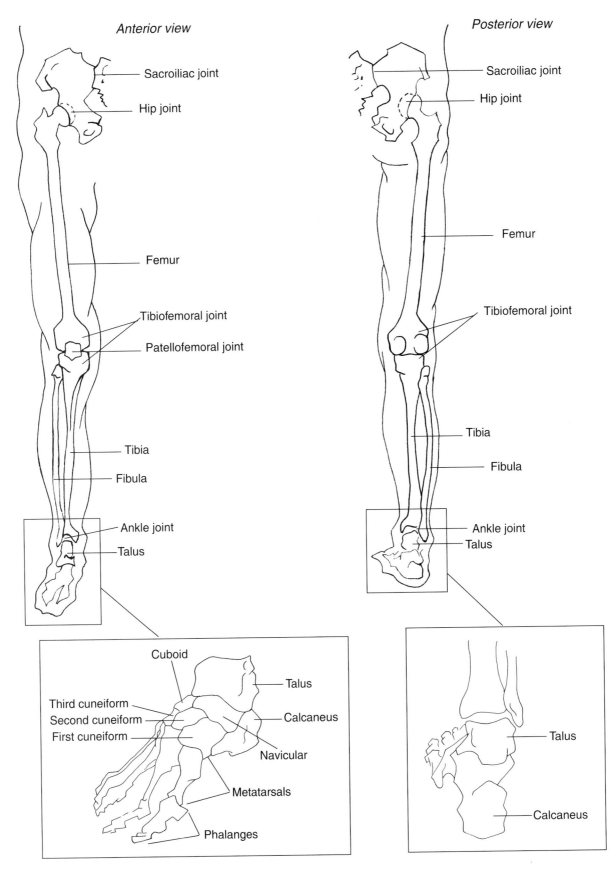

Figure 2.1 The lower kinetic chain.

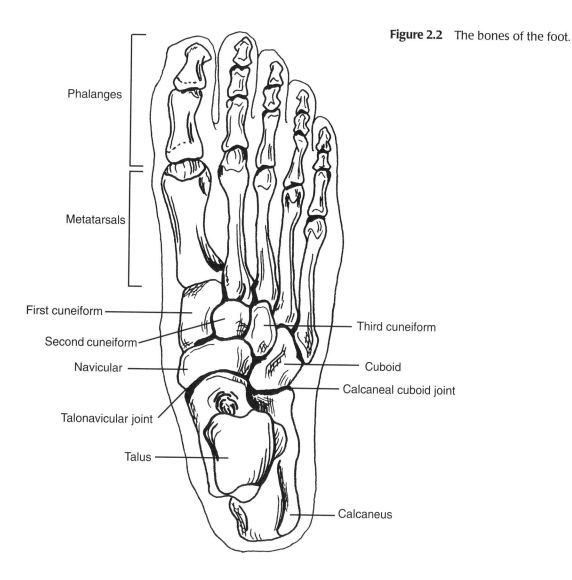

Figure 2.2 The bones of the foot.

Phalanges

Metatarsals

First cuneiform

Second cuneiform

Navicular

Talonavicular joint

Talus

Third cuneiform

Cuboid

Calcaneal cuboid joint

Calcaneus

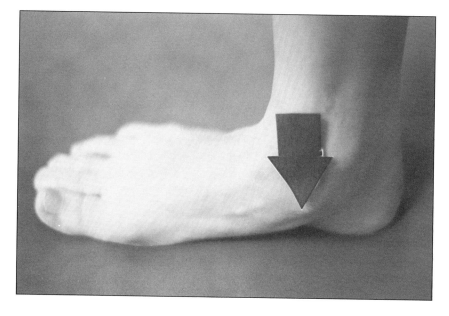

Figure 2.3 Foot in closed chain pronation.

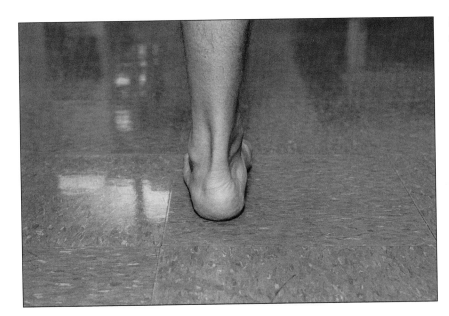

Figure 2.4 Foot in closed chain supination.

Effect on the Midtarsal Joint

The function of the midtarsal joint is an example of the old axiom of rehabilitation: "For distal mobility there needs to be proximal stability." The midtarsal joint, sometimes known as the transverse tarsal joint or Chopart's joint, is actually two joints, comprising the talonavicular joint and the calcaneocuboid joint, which together form an S-shaped line when viewed from above (Reigger, 1988) (Figure 2.5). Midtarsal joint stability depends on the position of the subtalar joint. As the subtalar joint becomes pronated in the closed chain position, the talus drops into an adducted and plantar flexed position (Vogelbach & Combs, 1987). This position allows more congruency of the articulations between the bones of the midtarsal joint. The long axes of the midtarsal joint become more parallel. Both of these adjustments allow more movement of the midtarsal joint. A pronated foot is often referred to as a "loose bag of bones" (Root et al., 1977).

With supination, the opposite configuration occurs. The talus abducts and dorsiflexes, making the joints of the midtarsal joint less congruent and the long axes of the bones more oblique. Less mobility results in the midtarsal area.

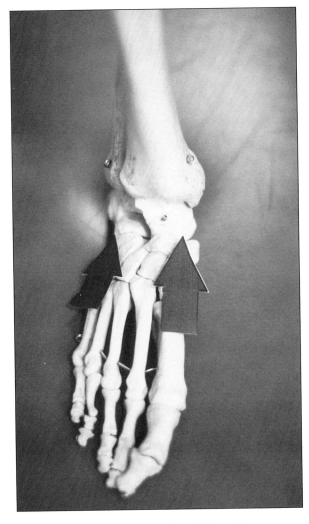

Figure 2.5 Midtarsal joint viewed from above.

Gait Cycle

The gait cycle may be divided into stance and swing phases (Figure 2.6). Approximately 60 percent of the gait cycle is spent in stance phase (Mann, 1982b). This phase lasts approximately .63 seconds (McPoil & Knecht, 1985; Murray, Drought, & Koury, 1964). Stance phase may be further divided into heel strike, midstance, and propulsion. At heel strike, the foot begins to pronate in order to adapt to the terrain. This pronation continues until the early part of midstance, when the foot begins to resupinate in order to provide a rigid lever from which to propel. Pronation usually takes only 25 percent of stance phase. Internal rotation of the tibia is complete at approximately the same time (Mann, 1982b). As explained later, prolonged or excessive pronation may adversely affect this internal rotation, leading to lower extremity problems.

Causes of Abnormal Pronation and Supination

Abnormal pronation and supination are compensatory mechanisms for anatomical problems. Many of these problems are abnormal osseous relationships, which result from faulty rotations in the lower extremity during embryological development (McPoil & Brocato, 1985). The most common is forefoot varus (Subotnick, 1975).

Forefoot varus is a bony abnormality in which the medial metatarsal heads are inverted or raised in relation to the plane of the calcaneus described by Root, Orien, and Weed in 1977, though the original paper on this topic was published by Hlavac in 1970 (Sims & Cavanagh, 1991). This condition may be viewed in subtalar neutral, as Figure 2.7 indicates. Most authors feel that forefoot varus is a congenital defect (Root et al., 1977). However, Jesse (1978) postulates that forefoot varus may also be caused by improper orthotic application in the correction of pronation or by a muscle imbalance between the anterior tibialis and peroneus longus. Whatever the cause, in weight-bearing stance and in propulsion, the medial aspect of the foot must contact the terrain surface. Pronation is the compensatory mechanism by which this contact occurs.

As for the prevalence of forefoot varus, Donatelli (1987) reports that for his patients it was the greatest cause of mechanical pain and dysfunction in the lower extremity. In a 1988 study by Donatelli, Hurlbert, Conaway, and St. Pierre, 95 percent of the patients demonstrated a forefoot varus. Schuster (1972) states that a large majority of the runners he treated demonstrated a moderate to severe forefoot varus, a much higher percentage than among his other patients.

Forefoot valgus is the opposite forefoot abnormality. Due to faulty embryological rotation, the metatarsal heads on the lateral aspect of the forefoot are higher than the medial metatarsal heads

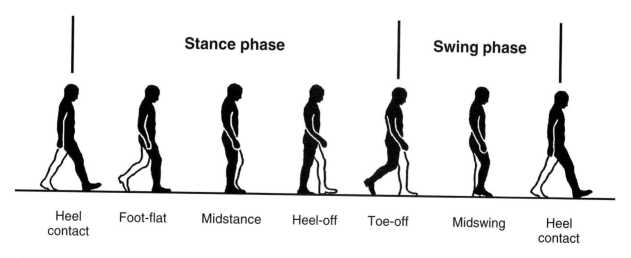

Stance phase   **Swing phase**

Heel contact   Foot-flat   Midstance   Heel-off   Toe-off   Midswing   Heel contact

Figure 2.6 The gait cycle.

From P. Allard, I. Stokes, and J-P. Blanchi, *Three-Dimensional Analysis of Human Movement*, 1995, Human Kinetics. Reprinted with permission.

(Figure 2.8). This eversion of the forefoot may involve all the metatarsals or only metatarsals 1 and 5, with metatarsals 2 to 4 in a varus or neutral attitude (Schoenhaus & Jay, 1980). The eversion creates a need for subtalar supination in order to bring the lateral aspect of the forefoot to the terrain surface.

The incidence of forefoot valgus is a source of debate. In a study of 276 patients, Burns (1977) found that 70.8 percent had forefoot valgus. He contends that many clinicians looking at the forefoot-rearfoot relationship measure incorrectly due to three reasons: (1) the examiner's predisposition to think that forefoot varus is the problem, (2) normal variation of neutral subtalar from the classic 2:1 ratio (see chapter 4), and (3) poor bisection of the posterior aspect of the heel.

Forefoot problems are not the only cause of abnormal compensation by subtalar joint pronation. Others include plantar flexed first ray, rearfoot varus, ankle joint equinus, and tibial varum (Root et al., 1977).

Listing the five most frequent reasons for abnormal pronation, Ramig, Shadle, Watkins, Cavolo, and Kreutzberg (1980) cite the following:

- Forefoot varus
- Rearfoot varus
- Short leg syndrome
- Leg length discrepancy
- External limb rotation

Halbach (1981) states that pronation may occur as a result of muscle imbalance among the foot's dynamic components, in which case these stabilizers are the key to rehabilitation of pronation-related problems. In this scenario, weakening of the dynamic supinators of the foot results in a hypermobile foot, which pronates.

Effects of Subtalar Pronation and Supination on the Distal Segments of the Lower Extremity

The "locking and unlocking" of the midtarsal joint through pronation and supination affects the proximal and distal mechanics of the lower extremity (McPoil & Knecht, 1985). For example, as pronation allows more motion of the midtarsal joint, the lesser tarsal bones, including the cuboid, become more mobile. As the midtarsal joint loosens during pronation, the mobile cuboid ceases to function efficiently as a pulley for the peroneus longus tendon as it crosses the foot to stabilize the first ray. With

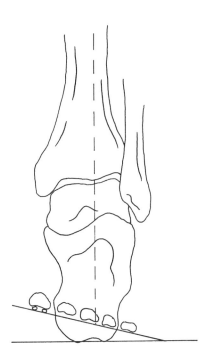

Figure 2.7 Forefoot varus.

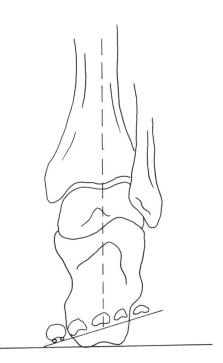

Figure 2.8 Forefoot valgus.

pronation there is a greater mobility of the first ray. Hypermobility of the first ray often leads to increased stress on the second metatarsal and/or a splaying apart of the metatarsal heads, either of which can cause symptoms such as bunions or neuromas and stress fractures (Root et al., 1977) (Figure 2.9).

Effects on the Tibia

There is an intimate relationship between the talus and tibia. Foot pronation with adduction of the talus is synchronous with internal rotation, medial deviation, and forward inclination of the tibia (Copland, 1989; McPoil & Knecht, 1985; Mann, 1982a; Oatis, 1988). Pronation tends to flex the knee, and supination tends to extend it, as can be demonstrated by lightly placing weight on one foot while rotating the calf to that side. As the tibia externally rotates, the arch on that side rises and weight is shifted to the lateral aspect of the foot, indicating a more supinated position. This motion also produces knee extension on that side (Figure 2.10).

Rotation as the main motion in the subtalar joint was first identified by Hicks (1953; Mann, 1982a), who referred to the joint as an oblique hinge joint. Wright, Desal, and Henderson (1964) conclude that the subtalar joint plays a small but integral part in the motion between the foot and leg in stance phase, characterizing it as a universal-joint type of linkage between the foot and leg. Inman (1976) describes ambulation as a series of rotations as the body moves in space. These rotations pass down along the lower extremity to the subtalar joint, where they are reduced so that the foot does not rotate. Rotations of the tibia are transformed into triplane movements at the subtalar joint.

Because of the axial orientation of the subtalar joint, there is internal rotation of the leg with calcaneal eversion and a corresponding external rotation of the leg with calcaneal inversion (Mann, 1982a). Although these motions are usually thought of in a one-to-one ratio, Olerud and Rosendahl (1987) found an average of .44 degrees of external rotation for every degree of subtalar supination, which supports the notion of the subtalar complex acting as a universal joint or torque converter.

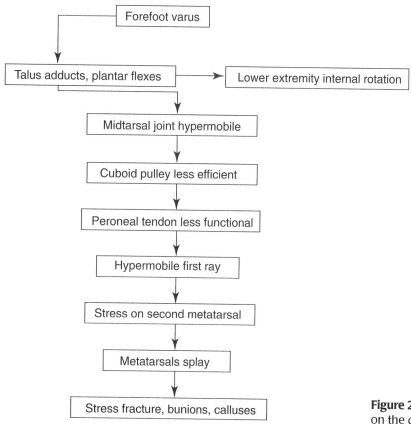

Figure 2.9　Effects of pronation on the distal extremity.

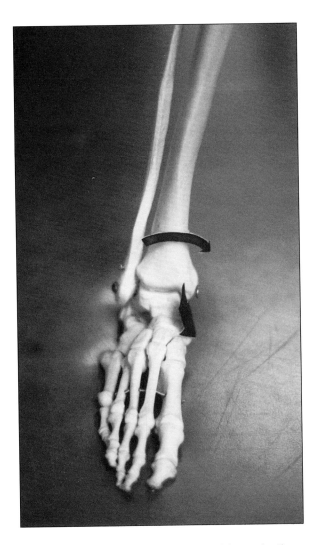

Figure 2.10 External rotation of the tibia, supination of the foot, and extension of the knee.

Lundberg et al. (1989) discount the idea that the talocalcaneal articulations are solely responsible for transfer of rotation, maintaining instead that all the joints distal to the talocrural joint have some function in the process. Their study showed an average of .2 degrees of tibial external rotation for each degree of subtalar supination. Levens, Inman, and Blosser (1948) determined that rotation of the tibia in relation to the floor was 7 degrees inward in the first part of stance phase and 8 degrees in the last part. This study also found that during walking, rotation around the vertical axis averaged 19.3 degrees at the lower leg. Copland (1989) found a significant difference in the amount of rotation of the tibia between pronating and normal

patients at 5 degrees of knee flexion. The average rotation for the normal group was 11.4 degrees versus 18.5 degrees for the pronating group. These studies indicate that there is a direct relationship between subtalar motion and rotation of the tibia. The following section examines the effect that this rotation may have on the knee.

Lower Extremity Rotation and Its Effect on the Knee

Abnormal pronation has been consistently mentioned as a possible source of knee dysfunction (Copland, 1989; D'Amico & Rubin, 1986; Donatelli, 1985; Halbach, 1981; Lattanza, Gray, & Kantner, 1988; Lutter, 1980; Mann, 1982a; Nesbitt, 1992; Ramig et al., 1980; Rodgers, 1988; Schuster, 1972). Many of these same authors have advocated foot orthotics as a treatment option for knee pain. Few authors, however, have attempted to establish the exact means by which foot mechanics adversely affect the knee.

Malalignment of the lower extremity is commonly blamed for knee problems (Reider, Marshall, & Warren, 1981). Increased Q angle, which creates a lateral pull of the quadriceps on the patella, is frequently mentioned as the culprit. The Q angle, as shown in Figure 2.11, is found by drawing a line from the anterior superior iliac spine and from the tibial tubercle to the midpoint of the patella (Buchbinder, Napora, & Biggs, 1979; Copland, 1989; D'Amico & Rubin, 1986; Ficat & Hungerford, 1979). Hossler and Maffei (1990) report that the approximate values for weightbearing and non-weightbearing Q angles in males are 15 and 10 degrees, respectively. In females these values are 20 and 15 degrees.

Pronation produces prolonged internal rotation of the leg and may force the patella laterally from the femoral groove (Ramig et al., 1980). This lateral riding of the patella then irritates the articular cartilage. Once osteochondral defects are present, no treatment will suffice except correcting the foot deformity. Pronation also increases internal tibial torsion, which in turn stresses the medial side of the knee. Lutter (1980) contends that a cavus or supinated foot never unlocks, which increases stress on the lateral aspect of the foot and knee. Supination also produces a varus moment at the knee.

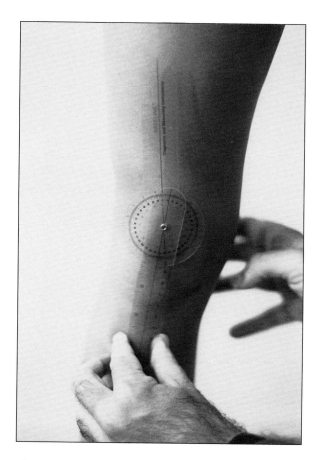

Figure 2.11   Q angle.

According to one theoretical model, Q angle decreases with pronation and increased internal rotation of the leg (Tiberio, 1987, 1988). In this view, pronation delays external rotation of the lower leg, which is a normal result of foot supination. External rotation is needed for extension of the knee. This external rotation is known as the "screw home" mechanism (Massie & Spiker, 1990; Sims & Cavanagh, 1991). Prolonged pronation of the foot requires compensation for the lack of external rotation of the tibia so that the knee may extend normally. Because the tibia does not rotate externally with prolonged pronation, internal rotation of the femur is the likely substitute. This type of rotation creates an increased force between the lateral aspect of the patella and the lateral femoral condyle.

This theory is partially substantiated in a study by Moss, DeVita, and Dawson (1992), which analyzed 44 high school runners in an attempt to formulate a predictive equation to screen patients for development of patellofemoral stress syndrome.

In this study the time to maximum pronation nearly coincided with the time to minimum Q angle. Normal biomechanics of the foot and ankle would have the leg starting external rotation as the foot begins to resupinate, and this external rotation should lead to an increasing Q angle. These authors theorize that if maximum pronation and minimum Q angle do not occur simultaneously as the biomechanics dictate, then rotational forces are acting in different directions at the knee, which could result in pathology at these sites.

This phenomenon is much greater when subtalar joint pronation occurs at midstance, where the joint normally should be supinating. Certain anatomical factors, such as femoral anteversion, may also accentuate these symptoms. Symptoms may occur anywhere in the lower extremity, most likely where there is a predisposing factor such as anatomical anomalies, weakness, or trauma. Other authors have found that when the lower extremity is subjected to the greater forces of running, very small deviations from normal may lead to lower extremity injury (Drez, 1982; Mann, 1982b).

Internal rotation of the tibia interferes with the normal knee-muscle force vectors, according to Beckman (1980). By shifting the patella medially, internal rotation increases the vertical pull of the vastus medialis obliques (VMO) while the medial pull is decreased. Beckman further states that orthotics reduce symptoms by two routes. First, they place the foot in a more neutral position, thereby decreasing the pronation that leads to excessive internal rotation of the tibia. This reduction of internal rotation prevents the decrease in the medial vector strength of the VMO. Second, by supinating the foot, orthotics encourage knee extension, which increases the stability of the knee and decreases the compressive forces on the knee.

As the tibia internally rotates with pronation, the femur internally rotates with greater excursion than the tibia, carrying the patella with it (D'Amico & Rubin, 1986). This medial shift of the patella then increases the Q angle, causing excessive lateral pressure and malalignment syndromes.

Copland (1989) theorizes that excessive pronation causes prolonged internal rotation of the tibia at midstance. With this internal rotation occurring at the same time the femur is externally rotating, the result is stress to the structures of the knee that limit knee rotation.

These theories are summarized in Figure 2.12.

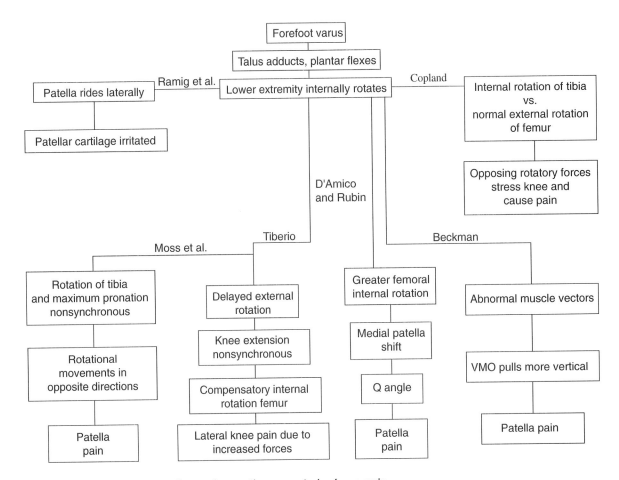

Figure 2.12   Theories of the effects of pronation on anterior knee pain.

Knee Injuries

The foregoing theoretically defined mechanisms explain why treatments involving foot biomechanics may benefit knee problems.

Chondromalacia Patellae and Patellofemoral Pain Syndrome

Chondromalacia patellae and patellofemoral pain syndrome, terms that are often used interchangeably, describe a condition in which there is a pathological degeneration of the articular cartilage of either the patella or the femur. Souza (1991) lists six common signs of this condition:

- Aching of the anterior aspect of the knee
- Giving way in near full extension
- Locking, stiffness, swelling, or popping
- Quadriceps atrophy
- Apprehension sign
- Crepitus

Chondromalacia patellae or anterior patellofemoral pain syndrome is frequently treated with orthotic therapy (Lutter, 1980). By reducing the pronatory forces that cause internal rotation of the tibia, orthotics may alter the biomechanics that adversely affect the knee. An orthotic may decrease the lateral pressure on the patella by reducing the compensatory internal rotation of the femur, as theorized by Tiberio (1987). A similar mechanism with different results is suggested by D'Amico and Rubin (1986), who speculate that by reducing the compensatory internal rotation of the femur in response to tibial internal rotation, orthotics reduce Q angle. Other possibilities are that foot orthotics, by reducing tibial internal rotation, may lead to decreased interference with the normal VMO vector force (Beckman, 1980) or to less lateral riding of the patella (Ramig et al., 1980). Either possibility relies on the fact that orthotics reduce tibial internal rotation in cases of excessive pronation.

Plica

Plica is another clinical entity that has been linked to pronation (Kergerris, Malone, & Johnson, 1988). A plica is a fold of knee synovium that is present in 20 to 60 percent of the population (Blackburn, Eiland, & Bandy, 1982). This synovial fold originates laterally at the quadriceps tendon on the superior aspect of the knee, then extends distally and medially to insert on the synovium of the infrapatellar fat pad. It is a normal structure but in cases of trauma, including high levels of activity, may become inflamed or thickened. In this condition, the fold may cause nonspecific patellofemoral pain as it passes back and forth over the femoral condyles. Weakness of the VMO may increase symptoms (Blackburn et al., 1982). A valgus knee position has also been implicated as a cause of irritation of this structure (Kergerris et al., 1988).

Orthotic therapy may reduce plica symptoms through the same mechanisms proposed for controlling chondromalacia symptoms or by reducing valgus malalignment at the knee. Another possibility is that decreased internal rotation of the tibia or decreased compensatory rotation of the femur may reduce the snapping or bowstring effect reported with plicas.

Patellar Tendonitis

Patellar tendonitis is also a common problem, especially in jumping athletes such as basketball players. It occurs at the insertion of the patellar tendon at the distal pole of the patella. Subotnick (1975) states that "abnormal rotation of the leg during compensatory foot movements" causes excessive tibial torsion. This torsion adversely affects the angle between the inferior pole and its attachment at the tibial tubercle. Orthotic therapy, by decreasing excessive pronation that leads to internal rotation of the tibia, may reduce torsion on the patellar tendon.

Iliotibial Band Syndrome

Iliotibial band syndrome is an overuse problem most often seen in athletes who train by running long distances. It is the most frequent problem associated with the lateral side of the knee (Clancy, 1980). Lutter (1981) states that iliotibial band syndrome is the hardest lower extremity problem to treat in runners. In his study of 836 runners with various lower extremity problems, he found that the average length of time away from full running was 90 days for iliotibial band syndrome. This syndrome was first described by Renne in 1975.

The iliotibial band originates from the pelvis as part of the gluteus maximus and the tensor fascia latae. It courses down the lateral thigh and inserts onto Gerdy's tubercle at the anterior lateral proximal tibia (Massie & Spiker, 1990). Iliotibial band syndrome problem is diagnosed by localizing pain on palpation at the lateral femoral condyle, where the tendon crosses over it. This area becomes inflamed as the tendon passes back and forth over the lateral femoral condyle.

Runners with cavus feet and varus knees have been reported to experience this syndrome more than others (Lindenberg, Pinshaw, & Noakes, 1984). Recovery may take almost two times as long for cavus-related iliotibial band syndrome as for pronation-related chondromalacia (Lutter, 1980). Iliotibial band syndrome is often experienced on the downhill leg of runners who favor one side of the road. It has been reported that patients respond to softer shoes (exerting less pronation control) and lateral heel wedges (pronating the foot slightly). Several of these details would indicate oversupination as a possible cause (Lindenberg et al., 1984).

It is difficult to visualize supination as a cause of iliotibial band syndrome based solely on the rotation of the tibia. Reducing supination and increasing pronation should lead to internal rotation of the tibia. The nature of the anatomy would appear to increase the tightness of the iliotibial band with pronation. Research indicates that the iliotibial band is not as taut in knee valgus as it is in varus (Lindenberg et al., 1984; Sutker, Jackson, & Pagliano, 1981). Lutter (1980) agrees that the greatest lower extremity problem occurring with the cavus foot is iliotibial band pain. He states that the midtarsal joint never unlocks to become supple. This lack of pronation increases the varus moment at the knee. Perhaps the reports of decreased iliotibial band symptoms with shoe changes and wedges are a result of decreased varus alignment rather than purely rotational changes.

Landry and Zebas (1985) postulate that the tensor fascia lata, by way of iliotibial band insertion, acts as an external rotator of the tibia. During excessive pronation, the iliotibial band may be overused to decelerate the internal rotation of the tibia. A study of running injuries by Macintyre, Taunton,

Clement, Lloyd-Smith, McKenzie, and Morrell (1991) revealed an increase of iliotibial band syndrome between 1981 (4.3 percent of patients) and 1980 to 1985 (7.5 percent). Their explanations for this increase included (1) increased sensitivity to the diagnosis; (2) antipronation shoes causing increased supination, resulting in increased tension on the iliotibial band; and (3) lateral breakdown in the shoe due to compression of the lower density foam.

Lower Leg Injuries

Shin splints and stress fractures are the two lower leg problems most commonly associated with pronation.

Shin Splints

Shin splints is a term frequently used for almost any pain in the lower leg. Unfortunately there are no set criteria for defining shin splints. Medial tibial pain along the proximal two-thirds of the bone is most often identified as shin splints (DeLacerda, 1980). Viitasalo and Kvist (1983) define shin splints as regular or long-lasting pain on the medial surface and distal two-thirds of the lower leg, without signs of a stress fracture. It also may be identified as anterior, posterior, or lateral shin or tibial pain (Massie & Spiker, 1990). Most authors blame shin splints on some type of overuse problem, particularly in runners.

Subotnick (1975) states that the anterior leg muscles (anterior tibialis, extensor digitorum longus, and extensor hallucis longus) are very susceptible to shin splint types of problems when they are overused to compensate for forefoot abnormalities. These muscles are active during toe-off, swing phase, and heel strike. Any use of these muscles during other parts of the gait cycle results in overuse and symptoms. With a forefoot varus, these anterior muscles must fire eccentrically to prevent foot slap. This firing out of phase results in stress and overuse. The major complaint with anterior shin splints is pain along the lateral border of the tibial crest. Tomaro, Rockar, Burdett, and Clemente (1992) treated 10 subjects with orthotics for lower leg symptoms. Electromyogram (EMG) studies with and without the orthotics revealed a significant increase in the duration of anterior tibialis activity following heel strike with the orthotics.

Another commonly identified form of shin splint is posterior compartment shin splints, characterized by pain along the posterior tibial border. The muscles in this area (posterior tibial, flexor digitorum longus, and flexor hallucis longus) are overused when prolonged pronation occurs during stance phase in an attempt to support the medial arch (McPoil & McGarvey, 1988). When running, this overuse may also occur during the first part of stance phase as the posteromedial muscle groups attempt to decelerate pronation (Landry & Zebas, 1985). Anderson (1990) believes that the posterior tibialis is the most important muscle in maintaining dynamic foot stability. As the posterior tibialis is stressed, it allows the foot to collapse into hyperpronation. Vogelbach and Combs (1987) believe that excessive pronation leads to fatigue of the posterior tibialis, which predisposes it to overuse types of problems. The etiology of the pain in this condition may reside in periostitis of the tibia, caused by abnormal pull from posterior tibial muscles, or it may be a compartment type problem (American Academy of Orthopedic Surgeons, 1991).

Any of these shin splints may occur due to overuse or training errors when combined with a biomechanical foot abnormality. Examples of training errors are sudden increases in mileage, changes in running surface (either from hard to soft, or vice versa), sudden increase in speed, and running on sloped surfaces (either on hills or sidehill running, as when running on a crowned road).

Stress Fractures

A problem frequently confused with shin splints is stress fracture of the lower leg. Most often the tibia rather than the fibula is involved with stress fractures (Davis, 1990). The incidence of stress fractures is on the increase, which may be due to increased athletic participation or better diagnostic capability (Jackson, 1991). Although overtraining is the major cause of stress fractures, several authors have reported increased stress fractures of the lower extremity secondary to faulty foot biomechanics (Milgrom et al., 1985; Myburgh, Grobler, & Noakes, 1988; Simkin, Leichter, Giladi, Stein, & Milgrom, 1989). Abnormal foot mechanics can cause stress to accumulate locally, which, combined with other faults such as overuse, creates a stressed area of bone. This area of stress has increased osteoclastic activity with normal osteoblastic activity. If the osteoblasts are not able to keep up with this osteoclastic activity, then a weakened area of bone results (Hughes, 1985). Initially the body responds with pain and inflammation. Eventually an area of callous will form (just as a regular fracture forms callous). Should the stress continue, the bone will eventually fracture, like a wire repeatedly bent in the same spot.

Most authors agree that rest is the major component of any treatment plan for a stress fracture. Orthotics may augment this treatment by placing the foot in a neutral position so that stress fractures will be minimized when the athlete returns to training (Milgrom et al., 1985).

Achilles Tendonitis

Achilles tendonitis is an inflammation of the common tendon of the posterior calf muscles. As the tendon passes down the leg, it rotates laterally upon itself. Pronation may accentuate this rotatory effect as the lower extremity is rotated (Davis, 1990). Especially susceptible is the area of the tendon 2 to 5 centimeters (1–2 in.) above the calcaneus, which has little blood supply. The rotatory effect may cause vascular impairment in this area. Clement, Taunton, and Smart (1984) attributed 56 percent of the cases of Achilles tendonitis they treated to hyperpronation.

Orthotics may reduce the symptoms of Achilles tendonitis by limiting pronation and thus limiting rotatory movement of the tendon at an area of poor blood supply. Orthotics may also act as a heel lift to reduce the tension on a tight heel cord. However, there is disagreement on the efficacy of orthotics. Dugas and D'Ambrosia (1991) state that orthotics are the primary method of treatment for injuries such as Achilles tendonitis, posterior tibial tendonitis, and plantar fasciitis, provided the cause was faulty biomechanics. This claim is contradicted by Lowdon, Bader, and Mowat (1984), who undertook a study of 33 sports-related cases of Achilles tendonitis. They implemented a program of ultrasound and exercise for one group of patients while ultrasound, exercises, and one of two foot orthotics (a viscoelastic heel lift or a sponge rub-ber heel pad) were given to the other two groups. All three groups showed some improvement, with the exercise and ultrasound only group improving the most. The authors speculate that the inserts did not significantly affect the outcome since simple heel lifts do not address pronation.

Foot Injuries

Foot biomechanics affect the lower leg and knee but may also cause symptoms in the foot, such as soft tissue or bony problems. Plantar fasciitis is the most common cause of foot pain in runners (Brody, 1980; Middleton & Kolodin, 1992). This term is often mistakenly used to describe pain anywhere on the bottom of the foot. It should be used to describe pain at the heel, near the insertion of the plantar fascia onto the calcaneus. The plantar fascia is a band of dense connective tissue that runs from the proximal phalanx of each toe to insert on the medial plantar aspect of the calcaneal tuberosity (Kosmahl & Kosmahl, 1987). The windlass effect, first described by Hicks (1954) and elaborated on by Dananberg (1986), involves the plantar aponeurosis lifting the arch during gait. As the great toe extends, the plantar aponeurosis is shortened, raising the arch and resupinating the foot. This repeated tugging at the plantar fascia may then cause microtrauma and inflammation at the insertion on the calcaneus or a bursitis (Robbins & Hanna, 1987). Often plantar fasciitis may be associated with a calcaneal spur.

The typical plantar fasciitis patient presents a classic description of the problem: Usually there is no trauma involved but a gradual increase in heel pain. The first few steps out of bed in the morning are the worst. With activity and as the day progresses, the pain decreases, but with overactivity the pain is exacerbated the next day. Standing after sitting for a prolonged period also is painful. Neale, Hooper, Clowes, and Whiting (1981) postulated that this pain upon weightbearing results from increased compartmental swelling, which puts pressure on local nerve fibers. With activity, this swelling is dissipated through the venous system.

Foot biomechanics related to overuse are frequently blamed for plantar fasciitis. Lutter (1981) and Newell (1977) state that plantar fasciitis occurs more frequently in rigid cavus feet. The cavus foot is unable to dissipate stress due to its rigid nature. Kosmahl and Kosmahl (1987) feel that excessive pronation leads to plantar fasciitis. As the calcaneus everts during pronation, the calcaneal tuberosity attachment of the plantar fascia is moved farther away from its distal attachment, increasing the tension at the calcaneus. Middleton and Kolodin (1992) state that a forefoot varus deformity may increase stress on the plantar fascia at its origin. They suggest six ways to treat plantar fasciitis:

- Stretching, proper warm up, and proper shoe selection
- Modalities
- Strengthening exercises
- Adhesive taping
- Orthotics
- NSAIDS and injections

Doxey (1987) advises that orthotics may prove beneficial for heel pain by

- decreasing abnormal compensatory mechanisms for malalignment,
- increasing the total contact area of the foot,
- providing relief at painful contact areas, and
- providing shock absorption.

Nesbitt (1992) observes that overpronation lowers the arch and stretches the plantar fascia. Conversely, high-arched feet also keep the plantar fascia under constant tension. An orthosis may be used to correct either condition and provide relief from plantar fasciitis.

A bunion is a deformity of the great toe in which the great toe takes a valgus position in relation to the metatarsal (Hunter, 1990). Subotnick (1975) blames the hypermobile pronated foot with forefoot varus as a frequent cause, advocating the use of functional control to prevent the progression of these deformities. Shaw (1975) states that a forefoot varus will cause the foot to enter the propulsive phase of gait everted and abducted. This position is mirrored by the hallux as the metatarsal adducts and dorsiflexes. The resulting deformity is a hallux valgus. Hlavac (1970) supports this etiology of bunions while noting that in the young, with good muscle power, hypermobile forefoot varus rarely causes problems. With fatigue or age, a dorsomedial bunion is a frequent finding for this type of foot. With a properly fitted

orthotic, the patient should ambulate more efficiently by bearing weight on the plantar aspect of the toe rather than pushing off medially and forcing the toe into abduction (Nesbitt, 1992). Hunter (1990) also feels that an orthotic may enhance weightbearing ability in a hypermobile first ray and thus prevent a bunion.

Summary

Pronation and supination are normal events within the gait cycle. When these events occur at the wrong time or in the wrong sequence, abnormal biomechanics may occur. Repetitive activities in which these abnormal biomechanics are utilized may lead to many of the injuries discussed in this chapter. Orthotic therapy may be of value in treating these injuries when improper pronation and supination are the cause.

References

American Academy of Orthopedic Surgeons. (1991). *Athletic training and sports medicine.* Park Ridge, IL: Author.

Anderson, E. (1990). The rheumatoid foot: A sideways look. *Annals of Rheumatic Diseases,* **49**, 851–857.

Beckman, S. (1980). Commentary on the foot and chondromalacia: A case of biomechanical uncertainty. *The Journal of Orthopaedic and Sports Physical Therapy,* **2**, 51–53.

Blackburn, T., Eiland, W., & Bandy, W. (1982). An introduction to the plica. *The Journal of Orthopaedic and Sports Physical Therapy,* **3**, 171–177.

Brody, D. (1980). Running injuries. *Clinical Symposia,* **32**, 1–37.

Buchbinder, M., Napora, N., & Biggs, E. (1979). The relationship of abnormal pronation to chondromalacia of the patella in distance runners. *Journal of the American Podiatry Association,* **69**, 159–161.

Burns, M. (1977). Non-weightbearing cast impressions for the construction of orthotic devices. *Journal of the American Podiatry Association,* **67**, 790–794.

Clancy, W. (1980). Runners injuries, part two: Evaluation and treatment of specific injuries. *The American Journal of Sports Medicine,* **8**, 287–289.

Clement, D., Taunton, J., & Smart, G. (1984). Achilles tendonitis and peritendonitis: Etiology and treatment. *American Journal of Sports Medicine*, **12**, 179–184.

Copland, J. (1989). Rotational motion of the knee. *Journal of Orthopaedic and Sports Physical Therapy*, **10**, 366–369.

D'Ambrosia, R., & Douglas, R. (1982). Orthotics. In R. D'Ambrosia & D. Drez (Eds.), *Prevention and treatment of running injuries* (pp. 155–164). Thorofare, NJ: Slack.

D'Amico, J., & Rubin, M. (1986). The influence of foot orthoses on quadriceps angle. *Journal of the American Podiatry Association*, **76**, 337–339.

Dananberg, H. (1986). Functional hallux limitus and its relationship to gait efficiency. *Journal of the American Podiatric Medical Association*, **76**, 648–650.

Davis, M. (1990). Rehabilitation of lower leg injuries. In W. Prentice (Ed.), *Rehabilitation techniques in sports medicine* (pp. 328–329). St. Louis: Times-Mirror/Mosby.

DeLacerda, F. (1980). Anatomical factors involved in shinsplints. *The Journal of Orthopaedic and Sports Physical Therapy*, **2**, 55–59.

Donatelli, R. (1985). Normal biomechanics of the foot and ankle. *The Journal of Orthopaedic and Sports Physical Therapy*, **7**, 91–95.

Donatelli, R. (1987). Abnormal biomechanics of the foot and ankle. *The Journal of Orthopaedic and Sports Physical Therapy*, **9**, 11–16.

Donatelli, R., Hurlbert, C., Conaway, D., & St. Pierre, R. (1988). Biomechanical foot orthotics: A retrospective study. *The Journal of Orthopaedic and Sports Physical Therapy*, **10**, 205–212.

Doxey, G. (1987). Calcaneal pain: A review of various disorders. *The Journal of Orthopaedic and Sports Physical Therapy*, **9**, 25–32.

Drez, D. (1982). Examination of the lower extremity in runners. In R. D'Ambrosia, & D. Drez (Eds.), *Prevention and treatment of running injuries* (pp. 15–19). Thorofare, NJ: Slack.

Dugas, R., & D'Ambrosia, R. (1991). Causes and treatment of common overuse injuries in runners. *Journal of Musculoskeletal Medicine*, **8**, 57–70.

Ficat, R., & Hungerford, D. (1979). *Disorders of the patellofemoral joint*. Baltimore: Williams & Wilkins.

Halbach, J. (1981). Pronated foot disorders. *Athletic Training*, **16**, 53–55.

Hicks, J. (1953). The mechanics of the foot. *Journal of Anatomy*, **87**, 345–355.

Hicks, J. (1954). The mechanics of the foot, part II: The plantar aponeurosis and the arch. *Journal of Anatomy*, **88**, 25.

Hlavac, H. (1970). Compensated forefoot varus. *Journal of the American Podiatry Association*, **60**, 229–233.

Hossler, P., & Maffei, P. (1990). Podiatric examination techniques for in the field assessments. *Athletic Training*, **25**, 311–317.

Hughes, L. (1985). Biomechanical analysis of the foot and ankle for predisposition to developing stress fractures. *The Journal of Orthopaedic and Sports Physical Therapy*, **7**, 96–101.

Hunter, S. (1990). Rehabilitation of foot injuries. In W. Prentice (Ed.), *Rehabilitation techniques in sports medicine* (pp. 342–357). St. Louis: Times-Mirror/Mosby.

Inman, V. (1976). *The joints of the ankle*. Baltimore: Williams & Wilkins.

Jackson, D. (1991). Stress fractures of the femur. *The Physician and Sportsmedicine*, **19**, 39–42.

Jesse, J. (1978). Orthotic misapplication, muscle imbalance and forefoot varus. *Journal of the American Podiatry Association*, **68**, 449–454.

Kergerris, S., Malone, T., & Johnson, F. (1988). The diagonal medial plica: An underestimated clinical entity. *The Journal of Orthopaedic and Sports Physical Therapy*, **9**, 305–309.

Kosmahl, E., & Kosmahl, H. (1987). Painful plantar heel, plantar fasciitis, and calcaneal spur: Etiology and treatment. *The Journal of Orthopaedic and Sports Physical Therapy*, **9**, 17–24.

Landry, M., & Zebas, C. (1985). Biomechanical principles in common running injuries. *Journal of the American Podiatric Medical Association*, **75**, 48–52.

Lattanza, L., Gray, G., & Kantner, R. (1988). Closed versus open chain measurements of subtalar joint eversion: Implications for clinical practice. *The Journal of Orthopaedic and Sports Physical Therapy*, **9**, 310–314.

Levens, A., Inman, V., & Blosser, J. (1948). Transverse rotation of the segments of the lower extremity in locomotion. *Journal of Bone and Joint Surgery*, **30**, 859–872.

Lindenberg, G., Pinshaw, R., & Noakes, T. (1984). Iliotibial band friction syndrome in runners. *The Physician and Sportsmedicine*, **12**, 118–130.

Lowdon, A., Bader, D., & Mowat, A. (1984). The effect of heel pads on the treatment of Achilles tendonitis: A double blind study. *The American Journal of Sports Medicine*, **12**, 431–435.

Lundberg, A., Svensson, O., Byland, C., Goldie, I., & Selvik, G. (1989). Kinematics of the ankle/foot complex, part 2: Pronation and supination. *Foot and Ankle*, **9**, 248–253.

Lutter, L. (1980). Foot related knee problems in the long distance runner. *Foot and Ankle*, **1**, 112–116.

Lutter, L. (1981). Cavus foot in runners. *Foot and Ankle*, **1**, 225–228.

Macintyre, J., Taunton, J., Clement, D., Lloyd-Smith, D., McKenzie, D., & Morrell, R. (1991). Running injuries: A clinical study of 4,173 cases. *Clinical Journal of Sports Medicine*, **1**, 81–86.

Mann, R. (1982a). Biomechanical approach to the treatment of foot problems. *Foot and Ankle*, **2**, 209–212.

Mann, R. (1982b). Biomechanics of running. In R. D'Ambrosia & D. Drez (Eds.), *Prevention and treatment of running injuries* (pp. 15–19). Thorofare, NJ: Slack.

Manter, J. (1941). Movements of the subtalar and tranverse tarsal joints. *Anatomical Record*, **80**, 397–410.

Massie, D., & Spiker, J. (1990). Foot biomechanics and the relationship to rehabilitation of lower extremity injuries. *Postgraduate Advances in Sports Medicine*, **1**, 1–11.

McPoil, T., & Brocato, R. (1985). The foot and ankle: Biomechanical evaluation and treatment. In J. Gould & G. Davies (Eds.), *Orthopedic and sports physical therapy* (pp. 300–341). St. Louis: Mosby.

McPoil, T., & Knecht, H. (1985). Biomechanics of the foot in walking: A functional approach. *The Journal of Orthopaedic and Sports Physical Therapy*, **7**, 69–72.

McPoil, T., & McGarvey, T. (1988). The foot in athletics. In G. Hunt (Ed.), *Physical therapy of the foot and ankle* (pp. 225–227). New York: Churchill Livingstone.

Middleton, J., & Kolodin, E. (1992). Plantar fasciitis: heel pain in athletes. *Athletic Training*, **27**, 70–75.

Milgrom, C., Giladi, M., Kashtan, H., Simkin, A., Chisin, R., Marguiles, J., Steinberg, R., Aharonson, Z., & Stein, M. (1985). A prospective study of the effect of a shock absorbing orthotic device on the incidence of stress fractures in military recruits. *Foot and Ankle*, **6**, 101–104.

Moss, R., DeVita, P., & Dawson, M. (1992). A biomechanical analysis of patellofemoral stress syndrome. *Athletic Training*, **27**, 64–67.

Murray, P., Drought, A., & Koury, R. (1964). Walking patterns of normal men. *Journal of Bone and Joint Surgery*, **46**, 335–354.

Myburgh, K., Grobler, N., & Noakes, T. (1988). Factors associated with shin soreness in athletes. *The Physician and Sportsmedicine*, **16**, 129–133.

Neale, D., Hooper, G., Clowes, C., & Whiting, M. (1981). Adult foot disorders. In D. Neale (Ed.), *Common foot disorders diagnosis and management: A general clinical guide* (pp. 56–57). New York: Churchill Livingstone.

Nesbitt, L. (1992). A practical guide to prescribing orthoses. *The Physician and Sportsmedicine*, **20**, 76–88.

Newell, S. (1977). Conservative treatment of plantar fasciitis. *The Physician and Sportsmedicine*, **5**, 68–73.

Oatis, C. (1988). Biomechanics of the foot and ankle under static conditions. *Physical Therapy*, **68**, 1815–1821.

Oledrud, C., & Rosendahl, Y. (1987). Torsion transmitting properties of the hindfoot. *Clinical Orthopedics*, **214**, 285–294.

Ramig, D., Shadle, J., Watkins, A., Cavolo, D., & Kreutzberg, J. (1980). The foot and sports medicine: Biomechanical foot faults as related to chondromalacia patellae. *The Journal of Orthopaedic and Sports Physical Therapy*, **2**, 48–50.

Reider, B., Marshall, J., & Warren, R. (1981). Clinical characteristics of patella disorders in young athletes. *American Journal of Sports Medicine*, **9**, 270–273.

Reigger, C. (1988). Anatomy of the foot and ankle. *Physical Therapy*, **68**, 1802–1804.

Renne, J. (1975). The iliotibial band friction syndrome. *Journal of Bone and Joint Surgery*, **57**, 1110–1111.

Robbins, S., & Hanna, A. (1987). Running related injury prevention through barefoot adaptations. *Medicine and Science in Sports*, **19**, 148–156.

Rodgers, M. (1988). Dynamic biomechanics of the normal foot and ankle during walking and running. *Physical Therapy*, **68**, 1822–1829.

Root, M., Orien, W., & Weed, J. (1977). *Clinical biomechanics: Vol. II. Normal and abnormal function of the foot.* Los Angeles: Clinical Biomechanics.

Schoenhaus, H., & Jay, R. (1980). Cavus deformities. *Journal of the American Podiatry Association*, **70**, 235–237.

Schuster, R. (1972). Podiatry and the foot of the athlete. *Journal of the American Podiatry Association*, **62**, 465–467.

Shaw, A. (1975). The effects of forefoot post on gait and function. *Journal of the American Podiatry Association*, **65**, 238–241.

Simkin, A., Leichter, I., Giladi, M., Stein, M., & Milgrom, C. (1989). Combined effect of foot arch structure and an orthotic device on stress fractures. *Foot and Ankle*, **10**, 25–29.

Sims, D., & Cavanagh, P. (1991). Selected foot mechanics related to the prescription of foot orthoses. In M.H. Jahss (Ed.), *Foot and ankle* (pp. 469–483). Philadelphia: Saunders.

Souza, D. (1991). Anatomy and pathomechanics of patellofemoral pain syndrome. *Postgraduate Studies in Sports Physical Therapy*, **1**, 1–8.

Subotnick, S. (1975). *Podiatric sports medicine.* Mt. Kisco, NY: Futura.

Sutker, A., Jackson, D., & Pagliano, J. (1981). Iliotibial band syndrome in distance runners. *The Physician and Sportsmedicine*, **9**, 69–73.

Tiberio, D. (1987). The effect of excessive subtalar joint pronation on patellofemoral mechanics: A theoretical model. *The Journal of Orthopaedic and Sports Physical Therapy*, **9**, 160–165.

Tiberio, D. (1988). Pathomechanics of structural foot deformities. *Physical Therapy*, **68**, 1840–1849.

Tomaro, J., Rockar, P., Burdett, R., & Clemente, F. (1992, June). The effects of foot orthotics on the EMG activity of selected leg muscles during gait. Paper presented at the meeting of the American Physical Therapy Association, Denver.

Viitasalo, S., & Kvist, M. (1983). Some biomechanical aspects of the foot and ankle in athletes with and without shin splints. *The American Journal of Sports Medicine*, **11**, 125–130.

Vogelbach, W., & Combs, L. (1987). A biomechanical approach to the management of chronic lower extremity pathologies as they relate to excessive pronation. *Athletic Training*, **22**, 6–16.

Wright, D., Desal, S., & Henderson, W. (1964). Action of the subtalar and ankle joint complex during the stance phase of gait. *Journal of Bone and Joint Surgery*, **46**, 361–382.

Orthotic and Related Research

3

Pronation and supination have been blamed for many maladies, and the use of orthotic therapy in the treatment of these problems has been controversial. Though the case for and against has been argued for years, good studies on the effectiveness of orthotics are hard to find. Few articles discuss how orthotics affect excessive movement but rather are discussions of subjective findings by the patient. This chapter will cover the most important literature on the pros and cons of orthotics as well as the various theories on why orthotics may work.

Early Orthotic Recommendations

Among the early advocates of orthotics, Schuster (1927) stated that orthotics redistribute weight over the plantar aspect of the foot.

Galland (1932) advocated a semirigid foot brace for the treatment of prolapse of the anterior and longitudinal arch.

In 1937, Fischer discussed the controversial nature of conservative treatment of flat foot and pes cavus. He stated that a support should have the following traits:

- Correction of heel pronation
- Correction of the reflection of the forefoot in standing
- Rigid support in the case of a mobile flat foot

The great foot physician Dudley J. Morton advised that patients try "compensatory insoles for pronated posture." His classic *Oh, Doctor! My Feet!* (1939), goes on to state that if the first metatarsal does not support enough weight, then three effects are noted:

- A double burden falls on the second metatarsal.
- The foot rolls inward to a pronated posture.
- An unnatural strain is placed on the muscles on the inner side of the ankle.

In *The Trainer's Bible* (1948), S.E. Bilk advocates sponge rubber arch supports for weakened arches and for the high-arched foot.

Recent Literature

Unfortunately, as time progressed, scientific data on the effects of orthotics did not significantly increase. Articles tended to emphasize subjective findings of the patient rather than observations of how orthotics affect excessive movement (Donatelli & Wooden, 1990). Many more of these advocate orthotics than criticize their use.

Flat Versus Cavus Feet as Injury Predictors

The relationship between foot types and injury is well documented in the running literature. Many authors agree that there is a direct correlation between high-arched, low-arched, pronated, or supinated feet and certain types of injuries.

James, Bates, and Osternig (1978) reviewed 180 patients with 232 orthopedic conditions, of whom 58 percent were found to have pronated feet, 20 percent had cavus feet, and 22 percent were considered neutral. No single diagnosis correlated with either pronation or supination. Lutter (1980) studied 213 runners with knee pain for four years: 77 percent had abnormal foot position (43 percent pronated, 34 percent of the cavus type). In the pronation group, problems included diffuse medial knee pain (57 percent), chondromalacia (28 percent), and medial joint pain (15 percent). Cavus problems were iliotibial band syndrome (25 percent) and lateral joint pain (9 percent).

Lutter (1981) also studied 836 runners with lower extremity injuries, of whom 9.6 percent had cavus feet. Most of the injuries were to the knee (57 percent), with the ankle-foot injuries tallying 38 percent. The length of time a runner was kept out of running was almost twice as long for a cavus foot as for a pronated foot.

In a retrospective study of 1,650 runners with various overuse problems, Clement (1981) found malalignment problems such as pronation in the majority. Subotnick (1981) observed that of 4,000 athletes seen in his office, 40 percent had flat feet, 20 to 25 percent had high arches, and 30 to 35 percent had normal arch height. D'Ambrosia and Douglas (1982) studied 50 runners with various orthopedic disorders, finding 44 percent had flat feet, 32 percent had high arches, and 24 percent normal arches. No specific diagnosis correlated with a certain arch type.

Powell, Kohl, Casperson, and Blair (1986), in a review of three epidemiological studies, concluded that the only established causative factor for running injuries was the number of miles run per week. Nevertheless, their paper states that "the hypothesis that structural abnormalities are a risk factor for running injuries is too reasonable to deny." Lysholm and Wiklander (1987) followed 55 running injuries in two clubs in Sweden for one year: 40 percent of the injuries involved intrinsic factors such as malalignment.

Pathological Conditions Resulting From Foot Types

Certain pathological conditions are reported as resulting from faulty foot mechanics.

Jernick and Heifitz (1979) found that chondromalacia was significantly correlated with increased pronation in 19 female runners.

DeLacerda (1980) found a significant correlation between shinsplints and an individual's navicular differential in a study of 81 female physical education class members. The navicular differential is a method of measuring pronation, obtained by measuring the height of the navicular tuberosity in a non-weightbearing position and subtracting the height of this landmark in a weightbearing position. Brody (1982) states that a navicular drop of 10 millimeters is normal but navicular drops greater than 15 millimeters are abnormal.

Low back pain has been correlated with pronation. Botte (1981) surveyed 25 hospital patients with low back pain as to foot type and pelvic imbalance. Nine patients had cavus feet, and 16 had pes planovalgus feet. He theorized that abnormal pronation may contribute to the development of low back pain by adding to the displacement of the sacroiliac joint.

Shin pain was positively correlated with pronation by Viitasalo and Kvist (1983), who found that patients with shinsplint symptoms had a longer time from heel strike to the maximum everted position, which indicates pronation.

Lindberg, Pinshaw, and Noakes (1984) blamed the cavus foot for iliotibial band syndrome.

Hughes (1985) studied 47 patients with metatarsal stress fractures for predisposing factors. Subjects with forefoot varus were found to be 8.3 times more likely to develop metatarsal stress fractures. Patients with decreased dorsiflexion were found to be 4.6 times more likely to sustain stress fractures.

Myburgh, Grobler, and Noakes (1988) studied 25 exercisers with shin soreness and 25 without shin soreness. They found a significant difference in the amount of subtalar and talar motion between the groups. As the motion increased, so did the chance of shin soreness. However, in subjects with unilateral pain, there was no difference in this range of motion between the symptomatic and asymptomatic legs.

Simkin, Leichter, Giladi, Stein, and Milgrom (1989) studied 295 military recruits to correlate arch type with stress fracture incidence. The study revealed that femoral and tibial stress fractures were more common with high-arched feet and that metatarsal stress fractures had higher incidence in feet with low arches.

Clanton (1989) states that subtalar instability may be the culprit in chronic ankle sprains where peroneal weakness, Achilles tightness, and proprioceptive dysfunction have been excluded.

Macintyre, Taunton, Clement, Lloyd-Smith, McKenzie, and Morrell (1991) did a retrospective study of 4,173 running injuries over a 4-year period, comparing the results to a previous study of 1,819 injuries by Clement (1981). Among the findings was an increase in iliotibial band friction syndrome, which was blamed on newer running footwear limiting pronation (resulting in a greater degree of supination or overcorrection of pronation).

Sammarco (1992) states that athletes with cavus feet are more likely to have a chronic Jones fracture, which is a fracture of the proximal fifth metatarsal that does not heal well. He notes that cavus feet are more rigid than flat feet and bear loads more on the lateral aspect of the foot.

Another interesting study involving navicular differential compared 50 patients with a history of a torn anterior cruciate ligament to 50 patients with intact anterior cruciate ligaments (Beckett, Massie, Bowers, & Stoll, 1992). The amount of navicular drop or pronation was significantly greater in the group with the torn anterior cruciate ligament.

Orthotic Therapy for Pathological Conditions

The effectiveness of orthotics in the treatment of anatomical anomalies and various disorders has also been scrutinized in the literature.

In the previously cited 1978 study of 180 runners by James et al., 83 pairs of orthotics (39 rigid, 44 flexible) were used to treat various lower extremity problems: 78 percent of the patients reported beneficial results. Bates, Osternig, Mason, and James (1979) filmed six runners from this study using three conditions: barefoot, with shoe, and with shoe and orthotic. The amount of pronation and length of pronated time were reduced significantly by the use of the orthotic device.

In a study of viscoelastic shoe inserts, Voloshin and Wosk (1981) found that viscoelastic material reduced shock waves to the musculoskeletal system by 42 percent. Sixty patients with degenerative joint disease of the ankle, knee, low back, or neck were also treated with viscoelastic inserts. For 78 percent of these, symptoms disappeared

completely, while 17 percent exhibited satisfactory improvement.

Scranton, Pedegana, and Whitesel (1982) studied the effects of low-dye taping, heel cups, and medial arch supports on momentary distribution of forces under the foot. Low-dye taping and heel cups diminished the duration of forces under the midfoot. Arch supports shifted the concentration of forces laterally but did not diminish their duration.

D'Ambrosia and Douglas (1982) found 72 percent in a group of 50 runners with various orthopedic disorders reporting improvement with orthotics. Of the 28 percent with no relief or worsened problems, a significant number had cavus feet, leading the authors to conclude that orthotic use was more appropriate for flat feet than cavus feet.

Sperryn and Restan (1983) studied 50 athletes with a variety of resistant symptoms including anterior knee pain, ankle pain, chronic sprains, and Achilles pain. Rigid orthoses (Rohadur) were given to 60 percent of these runners, while 32 percent received soft orthotics (cork and latex), 6 percent received both types, and 2 percent received heel lifts. Results over a 3 1/2-year period showed symptom relief in 56 percent of the patients and improvement in 8 percent. The remaining patients were distributed as follows: 14 percent reported no change, 6 percent could not tolerate the appliance, and 16 percent were lost to follow up. At the end of the study, 54 percent of the patients were still using their orthosis.

Milgrom et al. (1985) did a prospective study of 295 military recruits to see the effect of orthotic use on the incidence of stress fractures. One group of 143 members received military-issue stress orthotics made of PPT; the rest of the trainees wore military boots without orthotics. Overall, 31 percent of the recruits were diagnosed as having stress fractures during the 14-week training period. The incidence of metatarsal, tibial, and femoral stress fractures was reduced in the orthotic group, but only the incidence of femoral stress fractures was significant. The authors felt this finding was important since femoral stress fractures are more likely to displace than either tibial or metatarsal stress fractures.

D'Ambrosia (1980) treated 200 patients with orthotics over a 5-year period. The diagnoses included posterior tibial syndrome (most common), pes planovalgum metatarsalgia, plantar fasciitis, calcaneal spur, iliotibial band syndrome, cavus foot, leg length discrepancy, chondromalacia patellae, Achilles tendonitis, and others. The most improvement was seen in the following groups: posterior tibial syndrome group (70 percent of men and 83 percent of women showed improvement), the pes planovalgum group (90 percent showed improvement), the metatarsalgia group (84 percent of men and 89 percent of women showed improvement), and the calcaneal spur/plantar fasciitis group (85 percent of men and 76 percent of women showed improvement). The least improvement was seen in the iliotibial band syndrome group (66 percent showed improvement) and the cavus foot group (25 percent showed improvement).

Blake and Denton (1985) did a retrospective study by questionnaire and telephone of 180 patients, 98 percent of whom had received a hard orthotic for treatment of a lower extremity problem. Follow up lasted approximately one year. In descending order of frequency, problems treated were plantar fasciitis, posterior tibial shinsplints, chondromalacia, medial quadriceps strain, and patellar tendonitis. In this survey, 33 percent of the patients obtained complete relief. Half of the patients (including the preceding) obtained at least 90 percent relief, while nine out of ten obtained at least 50 percent relief. Other interesting statistics from this study include the following:

- 83 percent of the patients felt the orthotics were worth the expense.

- 40 percent had a problem with fitting.

- 75 percent felt that the orthotics improved their running.

Dugan and D'Ambrosia (1986), in another retrospective study, found orthotics improved the symptoms of 84 percent of 152 runners. These runners were classed as having posterior tibial syndrome, pes planovalgus, metatarsalgia, plantar fasciitis, cavus foot deformity, iliotibial band syndrome, calcaneal spurs, leg length inequality, chondromalacia patellae, or Achilles tendonitis. Half of these runners reported that they were able to return to prior levels of function without symptoms. Half of the patients who reported no relief had ill-fitting orthotics and 40 percent had cavus feet.

Smith, Clarke, Hamill, and Santopietro (1986) filmed 11 trained runners with and without soft and semirigid orthotics. The results showed that

soft and semirigid orthotics reduced rearfoot eversion movement by one degree (9 percent) compared to the control and reduced the speed of rearfoot eversion by 15 percent.

D'Amico and Rubin (1986) examined 21 patients standing with and without their orthotic devices. Eighteen of these patients had a decrease in their Q angle while standing in their orthotic. The average amount of the Q angle reduction was 6 degrees.

Riegler (1987) studied the use of semiflexible, thermoplastic, stance-molded orthotics in 235 patients with problems such as pronation, metatarsalgia, anterior knee pain, back pain, neuroma, and plantar fasciitis. Of these, 20.5 percent reported 100% improvement, 29.5 percent reported 75% improvement, 29.5 percent reported 50% improvement, 13.6 percent reported 25% improvement, and 6 percent reported no improvement.

Donatelli, Hulbert, Conaway, and St. Pierre (1988) administered questionnaires to 53 patients to determine the effectiveness of orthotic therapy. The most common deformity treated was forefoot varus. The most frequent reasons for orthotic therapy were foot pain (39 percent) and knee pain (31 percent). Overall, 96 percent reported pain relief from the orthotics; 94 percent were still wearing the orthotic at the time of the survey. Half reported they would not leave home without the orthotic.

Simkin et al. (1989) looked at arch type in relation to the use of orthotics for reducing stress fractures. Orthotic use reduced only the incidence of femoral stress fractures in the presence of high arches. The incidence of metatarsal stress fractures was reduced with orthotics only in low-arched feet. The incidence of tibial stress fractures was not affected by the use of an orthotic device.

Leard, Vogelbach, Gotwalt, Spiker, and Bowers (1989) reduced the average weightbearing talar tilt in 20 sprained ankles from 1.67 degrees to .69 degrees with the use of orthotics.

Holmes and Timmerman (1990) found that a simple metatarsal pad reduced metatarsal peak pressures 12 to 60 percent in females. Results varied in males.

Gross, Davlin, and Evanski (1991) sent questionnaires to current or prior orthotic users who were also runners with lower extremity problems. Of the 347 runners who answered the questionnaire, 30.8 percent reported complete relief of symptoms, 44.7 percent great improvement,

15.8 percent slight improvement, 7.5 percent no improvement, and 1.2 percent got worse. Distribution of orthotic types was 63 percent flexible, 23 percent semirigid, and 14 percent rigid.

Tristant and Blake (1991) theorized that functional orthotic devices were more effective on excess calcaneal motion than on extrinsically caused motions. They found that subjects tended to have more calcaneal varus when running than walking. From this they concluded that orthotics tend to work better in controlling varus during running than during walking.

Greenberg, Sanderson, Taunton, and Macintyre (1991) studied 13 skiers, divided according to standard versus custom-molded ski boot footbeds. The group fitted with custom cork footbeds showed a significant reduction in motion of the navicular, decreased rearfoot angle, and significant realignment of the tibial tuberosity. The authors concluded that custom-molded ski boot footbeds improved the neutral position of the foot and controlled subtalar motion better than regular footbeds.

Orteza, Vogelbach, and Denegar (1992) studied the effects of orthotics on pain and balance in patients who had sprained an ankle. Subjects were divided into two groups (injured and postinjury), and three conditions were tested: molded orthotic of Aquaplast, nonmolded orthotic of Plastazote, and no orthotic. Molded orthotics significantly improved the balance of the postinjury group and decreased pain during jogging for the injured group. There was no significant improvement in the nonmolded orthotic group or in the group with no orthotics.

Articles Citing Contraindications to Orthotic Therapy

Not all research supports the premise that foot types are correlated with injuries. The effects of orthotics are also questioned in several articles in the literature.

Early opponents to foot supports include Bankart (1935), who opposed the use of any type of support. Bilk (1948) stated that rigid steel arch supports have no place in athletics. Jesse (1978) theorized that one cause of forefoot varus was the improper use of orthotic devices to treat pronated feet, citing several studies linking correction of valgus calcaneus with the formation of forefoot varus. Penneau, Lutter, and Winter (1982), study-

ing children with pes planus, found no significant radiological difference among these conditions: barefoot, Thomas heel, over-the-counter inserts, and molded orthotic.

One of the more widely quoted studies on orthotic efficacy is by Rodgers and LeVeau (1982), who used slow-motion filming to show no significant differences in the amount of pronation with and without orthotics.

D'Ambrosia and Douglas (1982) state that orthotics that are worn constantly may cause muscles and ligaments around joints to become weakened due to disuse. They advocate that orthotics be worn only during times of severe or repeated stress.

Gill (1985) questions the costs of orthotics versus the results they give. He advises anyone investing in orthotics not to expect any miracles. He calls orthotics aids, not cure-alls.

Peter Cavanagh, professor of biomechanics at Pennsylvania State University, University Park, as quoted in an article by Murphy (1986), believes that orthoses are only effective for the recreational runner. He states that the competitive runner, rather than having something extra or loose in the shoe, should have only the support built into the shoe.

Warren and Jones (1987) studied variables in 91 runners in order to find a predictor for plantar fasciitis, past or present. They concluded that variables such as leg length inequality, dorsiflexion ability, ankle flexibility, arch height, pronation while running, body characteristics, age, time of foot contact, and type of foot strike had no significant predictive value for plantar fasciitis.

Another study on the predictability of running injuries focused on 134 runners with running-related injuries, using 72 anatomical variables (Warren & Davis, 1988). The variables were placed into six factor groups: spine, hip, knee, ankle, subtalar, and midtarsal. The subtalar joint exam included supination, pronation, and neutral varus and valgus. The midtarsal joint exam included varus and valgus movement, tibial varus, and range of the first ray. The conclusion of this study was that none of the factors was a good predictor of running pain.

Milgrom, Burr, Boyd, Robin, Higgins, and Radin (1990) found no significant difference in the incidence of tibial stress fractures with and without viscoelastic orthotics in the canine animal model.

Giladi, Milgrom, and Simkin (1991) studied stress fractures of the tibia and femur in 312 military recruits. The only significant variables were narrower tibiae and a higher degree of external rotation. Hindfoot eversion-inversion from neutral subtalar position was not a significant factor.

Moss, DeVita, and Dawson (1992) studied 29 subjects to test the effect of certain anthropometric, strength, and kinematic variables on patellofemoral stress syndrome. No significant difference was found between the symptomatic and asymptomatic groups in either degree of maximum pronation or time to maximum pronation.

Summary

Scientific studies and arguments both support and question anatomical foot and arch differences as the cause of lower extremity problems. There is also disagreement on the effectiveness of orthotics in treating many of these same maladies. Most researchers feel that orthotics provide some type of biomechanical answer to a wide range of lower extremity problems, although the mechanism is subject to debate. Some researchers have found that orthotics are not beneficial.

The truth may lie somewhere between the two points of view. Steven Subotnick has said (as quoted by Murphy, 1986), "Orthoses are not a panacea, but are only part of the overall solution." He also states that orthoses are overprescribed, poorly understood, and usually not fully integrated into a complete treatment plan with full rehabilitation (1983). Regardless of the neutrality of the foot as it ambulates, the body cannot take the abuses of overtraining and overuse.

References

Bankart, A. (1935). The treatment of minor maladies of the foot. *Lancet*, **1**, 249.

Bates, B., Osternig, L., Mason, B., & James, L. (1979). Foot orthotic devices to modify selected aspects of lower extremity mechanics. *The American Journal of Sports Medicine*, **7**, 338–342.

Beckett, M., Massie, D., Bowers, K., & Stoll, D. (1992). Incidence of hyperpronation on the ACL injured knee: A clinical perspective. *Athletic Training*, **27**, 58–62.

Bilk, S. (1948). *The Trainers Bible* . New York: Reed.

Blake, R., & Denton, J. (1985). Functional foot orthoses for athletic injuries. *Journal of the American Podiatric Medical Association*, **75**, 359–362.

Botte, R. (1981). An interpretation of the pronation syndrome and foot types of patients with low back pain. *Journal of the American Podiatry Association*, **71**, 243–252.

Brody, D. (1982). Techniques in the evaluation and treatment of the injured runner. *Orthopedic Clinics of North America*, **13**, 541–558.

Clanton, T. (1989). Instability of the subtalar joint. *Orthopedic Clinics of North America*, **20**, 583–592.

Clement, D. (1981). A survey of overuse running injuries. *The Physician and Sportsmedicine*, **9**, 47–49.

D'Ambrosia, R. (1980). Orthotic devices in running injuries. *Clinics in Sports Medicine*, **4**, 611–618.

D'Ambrosia, R., & Douglas, R. (1982). Orthotics. In R. D'Ambrosia & D. Drez (Eds.), *Prevention and treatment of running injuries* (pp. 155–164). Thorofare, NJ: Slack.

D'Amico, J., & Rubin, M. (1986). The influence of foot orthotics on the quadriceps angle. *Journal of the American Podiatric Medical Association*, **76**, 337–339.

DeLacerda, F. (1980). A study of anatomical factors involved in shinsplints. *The Journal of Orthopaedic and Sports Physical Therapy*, **2**, 55–59.

Donatelli, R., Hurlbert, C., Conaway, D., & St. Pierre, R. (1988). Biomechanical foot orthotics: A retrospective study. *The Journal of Orthopaedic and Sports Physical Therapy*, **10**, 205–212.

Donatelli, R., & Wooden, M. (1990). Biomechanical orthotics. In R. Donatelli (Ed.), *The biomechanics of the foot and ankle* (pp. 193–216). Philadelphia: Davis.

Dugan, R., & D'Ambrosia, R. (1986). Proceedings of the sixteenth annual meeting. *Foot and Ankle*, **6**, 313.

Fischer, E. (1937). The use of mechanical support in the treatment of foot affections. *The Journal of Bone and Joint Surgery*, **19**, 185–194.

Galland, W. (1932). A semiflexible brace for the support of the longitudinal arch of the foot. *The American Journal of Surgery, 17,* 442–443.

Giladi, M., Milgrom, C., & Simkin, A. (1991). Stress fractures: Identifiable risk factors. *The American Journal of Sports Medicine, 19,* 647–652.

Gill, E. (1985, February). Orthotics. *Runner's World,* 55–57.

Greenberg, S., Sanderson, D., Taunton, J., & Macintyre, J. (1991). Control of subtalar motion with the use of ski boot footbeds. *Clinical Journal of Sports Medicine, 1,* 188–192.

Gross, M., Davlin, L., & Evanski, P. (1991). Effectiveness of orthotic shoe inserts in the long distance runner. *The American Journal of Sports Medicine, 19,* 409–411.

Holmes, G., & Timmerman, L. (1990). A quantitative assessment of the effect of metatarsal pads on plantar pressures. *Foot and Ankle, 11,* 141–145.

Hughes, L. (1985). Biomechanical analysis of the foot and ankle for predisposition to developing stress fractures. *The Journal of Orthopaedic and Sports Physical Therapy, 7,* 96–99.

James, S., Bates, B., & Osternig, L. (1978). Injuries to runners. *The American Journal of Sports Medicine, 6,* 40–49.

Jernick, S., & Heifitz, N. (1979). An investigation into the relationship of foot pronation to chondromalacia patellae. *Sports Medicine '79,* (p. 1). Mt. Kisco, NY: Futura.

Jesse, J. (1978). Orthotic misapplication, muscle imbalance and forefoot varus. *Journal of the American Podiatry Association, 68,* 449–454.

Leard, J., Vogelbach, W., Gotwalt, D., Spiker, J., & Bowers, K. (1989). Effects of neutral orthotics in the treatment of acutely sprained ankles. *Proceedings of the 1989 NATA Convention, 24,* 124.

Lindberg, G., Pinshaw, R., & Noakes, T. (1984). Iliotibial band syndrome in runners. *The Physician and Sportsmedicine, 12,* 118–130.

Lutter, L. (1980). Foot related knee problems in the long distance runner. *Foot and Ankle, 1,* 112–116.

Lutter, L. (1981). Cavus foot in runners. *Foot and Ankle, 1,* 225–228.

Lysholm, J., & Wiklander, J. (1987). Injuries in runners. *The American Journal of Sports Medicine, 15,* 168–170.

Macintyre, J., Taunton, J., Clement, D., Lloyd-Smith, D., McKenzie, D., & Morrell, R. (1991). Running injuries: A clinical study of 4,173 cases. *Clinical Journal of Sports Medicine, 1,* 81–86.

Milgrom, C., Burr, D., Boyd, R., Robin, G., Higgins, W., & Radin, E. (1990). The effect of a viscoelastic orthotic on the incidence of tibial stress fractures in an animal model. *Foot and Ankle, 10,* 276–279.

Milgrom, C., Giladi, M., Kashtan, H., Simkin, A., Chisin, R., Marguiles, J., Steinberg, R., Aharonson, Z., & Stein, M. (1985). A prospective study of the effect of a shock absorbing orthotic device on the incidence of stress fractures in military recruits. *Foot and Ankle, 6,* 101–104.

Morton, D. (1939). *Oh, Doctor! My Feet!* New York: Appleton-Century.

Moss, R., DeVita, P., & Dawson, M. (1992). A biomechanical analysis of patellofemoral stress syndrome. *Athletic Training, 27,* 64–67.

Murphy, P. (1986). Orthoses: Not the sole solution for running ailments. *The Physician and Sportsmedicine, 14,* 164–167.

Myburgh, K., Grobler, N., & Noakes, T. (1988). Factors associated with shin soreness in athletes. *The Physician and Sportsmedicine, 16,* 129–134.

Orteza, L., Vogelbach, W., & Denegar, C. (1992). The effect of molded and unmolded orthotics on balance and pain while jogging following inversion ankle sprain. *Athletic Training, 27,* 80–84.

Penneau, K., Lutter, L., & Winter, R. (1982). Pes planus: Radiographic changes with foot orthoses and shoes. *Foot and Ankle, 2,* 299–303.

Powell, E., Kohl, H., Casperson, C., & Blair, S. (1986). An epidemiological perspective on the causes of running injuries. *The Physician and Sportsmedicine, 14,* 100–114.

Riegler, H. (1987). Orthotic devices for the foot. *Orthopedic Review, 16,* 293–303.

Rodgers, M., & LeVeau, B. (1982). Effectiveness of foot orthotic devices used to modify pronation in runners. *The Journal of Orthopaedic and Sports Physical Therapy, 4,* 86–90.

Sammarco, G. (1992). Be alert for Jones fractures. *The Physician and Sportsmedicine*, **20**, 101–110.

Schuster, O. (1927). *Foot Orthopedics*. New York: Marbridge.

Scranton, P., Pedegana, L., & Whitesel, J. (1982). Gait analysis: Alterations in support phase forces using supportive devices. *The American Journal of Sports Medicine*, **10**, 6–10.

Simkin, S., Leichter, I., Giladi, M., Stein, M., & Milgrom, C. (1989). Combined effect of foot arch structure and an orthotic device on stress fractures. *Foot and Ankle*, **10**, 25–29.

Smith, L., Clarke, T., Hamill, C., & Santopietro, F. (1986). The effects of soft and semirigid orthoses upon rearfoot movement in running. *Journal of the American Podiatric Medical Association*, **76**, 227–233.

Sperryn, P., & Restan, L. (1983). Podiatry and the sports physician: An evaluation of orthoses. *British Journal of Sports Medicine*, **17**, 129–134.

Subotnick, S. (1981). The flat foot. *The Physician and Sportsmedicine*, **9**, 85–91.

Subotnick, S. (1983). Foot orthoses: An update. *The Physician and Sportsmedicine*, **11**, 103–109.

Tristant, S., & Blake, R. (1991). The myth of running limb varus. *Journal of the American Podiatric Medical Association*, **81**, 325–327.

Viitasalo, J., & Kvist, M. (1983). Some biomechanical aspects of the foot and ankle in athletes with and without shinsplints. *The American Journal of Sports Medicine*, **11**, 125.

Voloshin, A., & Wosk, J. (1981). Influence of artificial shock absorbers on human gait. *Clinical Orthopedics and Related Research*, **160**, 52–56.

Warren, B., & Davis, V. (1988). Determining predictor variables for running related pain. *Physical Therapy*, **68**, 647–651.

Warren, B., & Jones, J. (1987). Predicting plantar fasciitis. *Medicine and Science in Sports and Exercise*, **19**, 71–73.

Biomechanical Examination

4

This chapter introduces the concepts and skills needed to perform a clinical and biomechanical examination of the foot and ankle to determine if orthotic therapy should be included in an overall treatment plan. This discussion is not meant to be an all-inclusive examination of the lower kinetic chain; rather it is directed toward specific examination of the foot and ankle with regard to orthotic fabrication. We assume that additional examination techniques, such as manual muscle testing, leg length measurements, range of motion tests, evaluation of muscular tightness, and orthopedic assessment, are included in the examination as warranted.

Figure 4.1 is a sample form that could be used by the clinician to document the objective portion of the clinical examination. This form is adaptable to the needs of clinicians who primarily use the palpation method and observation techniques as well as those using goniometric methods. Data can be recorded by circling the appropriate icons representing the deformity, by filling in the appropriate spaces with goniometric measurements, or by using a combination of both methods. We encourage you to design your own work sheet for the clinical examination and orthotic fabrication, one that meets your specific needs.

Clinical Examination

The following sections represent the major portions of the physical and biomechanical examination of the patient.

History

The first part of the examination includes a detailed history of the patient's symptoms and activity levels. The history is especially important with an athlete in training because of the effect of repetitive training stress on the mechanics of the foot and ankle. Perhaps 60 percent of the injuries associated with runners are attributable to training errors (James, Bates, & Osternig, 1978). Examples of training errors include increase in mileage, increase in speed workouts, change of training surface, lack of or change in warm-up or cool-down routine, change in running shoes, and wearing out of training shoes. Questions to be asked during the history include the following:

- What brought on the pain?
- How long has the pain been present?
- What type of pain is it? Sharp, dull, aching, pins and needles, throbbing, numbness, tingling?
- Do you notice a change in temperature? Are your feet colder than normal?
- Is your pain present all the time? If not, what brings about your symptoms?
- Have you ever had a similar injury? If so, what did you do for it?
- Does anything relieve your symptoms?
- Is there a position or activity that makes the pain better or worse?
- Do you have a family history of arthritis, circulatory problems, diabetes, etc.?
- Have you seen a doctor or any other health care professional about this injury?

Figure 4.1 Biomechanical Examination Worksheet

Name _____   Date _____

History:_____
_____

Observation: _____
_____

Determination Neutral Subtalar Joint Position (NSTJP)
NSTJP = MAX. INVERSION + MAX. EVERSION = TOTAL ROM \3

Goniometric measurements	LEFT	RIGHT
Maximal inversion		
Maximal eversion		
Total ROM (INV + EVR)		
Neutral subtalar joint position		

Rearfoot Alignment with foot in NSTJP
(using goniometric or palpation technique)

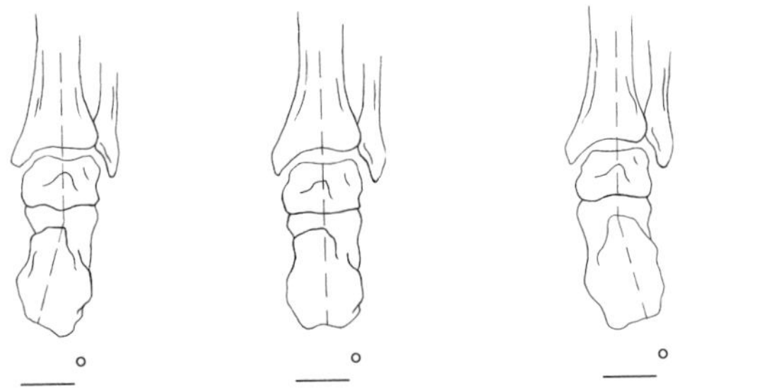

Forefoot Alignment

Varus   Neutral   Rearfoot Valgus   Varus   Neutral   Valgus

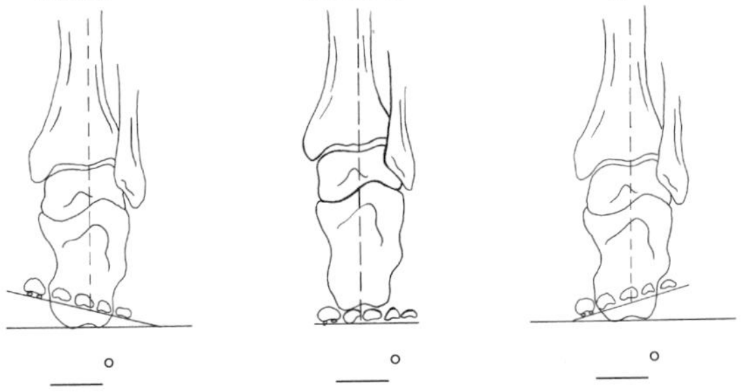

1st Ray Position

Dorsiflexed   Neutral   Plantar = flexed

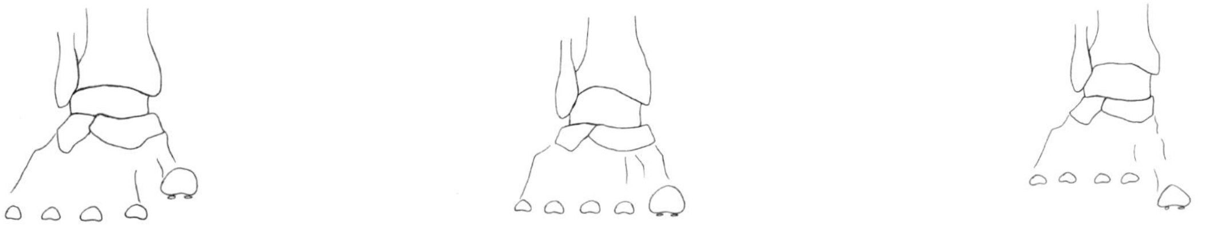

Goniometric measurements	LEFT	RIGHT
1st ray dorsiflexion/plantar flexion		
Ankle joint dorsiflexion (knee extended)		
Ankle joint dorsiflexion (knee flexed)		
Tibial varum/valgum		
Standing calcaneal		
Navicular differential		
Q angle		
A angle		

Summary of gait analysis:
_____

Shoe wear pattern:
_____

Orthotic prescription:

Questions Specifically for Athletes

- What type of training do you do? (speed, intervals, fartlek)
- How often do you run?
- How many miles per week do you run?
- Have you recently changed any part of your training?
- What type of surface do you run on?
- Have you changed to a new running shoe recently?
- What type of warm-up and cool-down do you perform?
- Is there anything else you would like to tell me about your injury that you think is important?

Observation

For observation, patients should stand in a relaxed position, wearing shorts but with their shoes and socks removed (see Figure 4.2). They should be observed in the frontal and sagittal planes (see Figure 4.3) from the anterior, posterior, and lateral directions for the following lower extremity conditions and alignments:

- Spinal curvatures
- Pelvic tilt
- Femoral neck anteversion or retroversion
- Patellar position, patella squinting, alta, etc.
- Alignment of lower extremity with regard to varus, valgum, or recuvatum of the knees
- Internal or external tibial rotation
- Pronation or supination
- Retrocalcaneal exostosis (pump bumps)
- Medial bulging of the talus and navicular
- Hallux valgus
- Toe position and alignment
- Hammer toes or claw toes
- Callus formation (Figure 4.4)

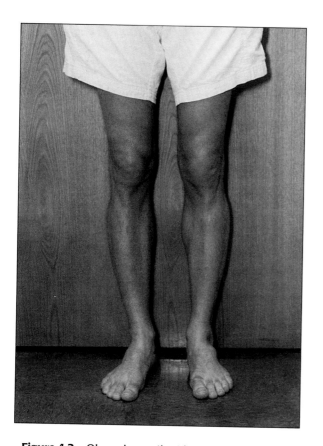

Figure 4.2 Observing patient in standing position.

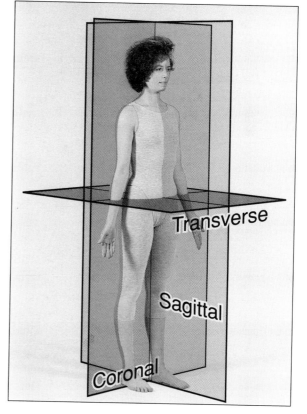

Figure 4.3 Cardinal planes of the body.
From D. Perrin, *Isokinetic Exercise and Assessment*, 1993, Human Kinetics. Reprinted by permission.

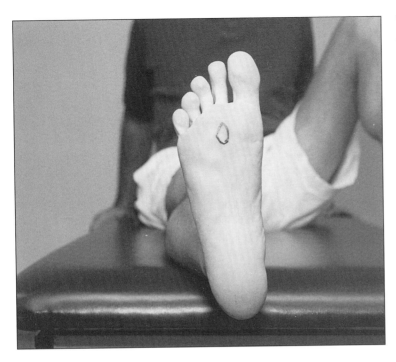

Figure 4.4   Observation of the plantar aspect of the foot for callus formation.

Objective Examination

The purpose of the objective examination is to systematically determine what if any structural or positional abnormalities are present in the patient. These abnormalities can be observed and in some cases measured by the clinician. This information is then used in determining the treatment protocol which may include orthotic intervention or other types of rehabilitative techniques.

Materials Needed

The following materials are needed for the objective examination:

- Felt tip marking pen
- Clear plastic goniometer with one degree increments

Patient Positioning

The patient is positioned prone on an examination table, with ankles extended approximately 6 inches over the edge. The calcaneus should be parallel to the table. This orientation is accomplished by flexing, abducting, and externally rotating the opposite limb as shown in Figure 4.5.

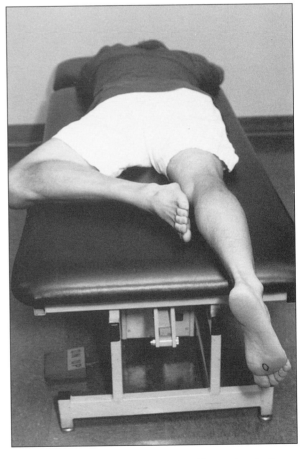

Figure 4.5   Patient positioning for biomechanical examination.

Lines of Bisection

With the patient positioned, two lines of bisection will be established as reference points for the goniometric measurements. The first line extends through the posterior aspect of the calcaneus, bisecting the calcaneus into left and right portions. To locate this line, palpate the calcaneus with the dorsal aspect of your index fingers and visualize the midline of the calcaneus, as illustrated in Figure 4.6. Place two dots on the calcaneus to represent the top and bottom of the line (Figure 4.7). The second line of bisection will split the distal one-third of the lower leg, extending down the lower leg almost to the level of the Achilles tendon (however, when drawing the line, disregard the Achilles tendon). Place two or three dots along the lower leg, as illustrated in Figure 4.8. Now draw the two lines using a goniometer edge and marking pen as shown in Figure 4.9.

Determining Neutral Subtalar Joint Position

Determining neutral subtalar joint position is a critical step in the examination process and later in orthotic fabrication. Neutral subtalar joint position is the position of the foot in the midstance phase of the gait cycle where the foot is thought to function most efficiently. Osseus or positional deviations from this position can cause compensatory movements resulting in pathology to the lower kinetic chain. Root, Orien, Weed, and Hughes (1971) defined neutral subtalar joint position as the position in which the foot is neither pronated nor supinated. From this position, full supination of the normal subtalar joint inverts the calcaneus twice as many degrees as full pronation everts it, and the talus is congruent with the navicular (Root, Orien, & Weed, 1977) (Figure 4.10).

Drawing the Lines of Bisection

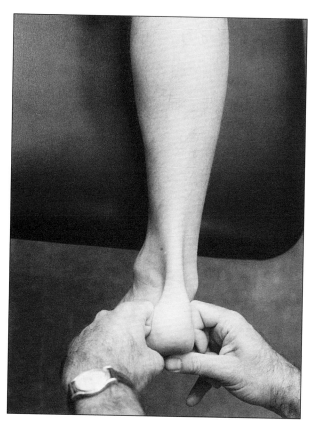

Figure 4.6 Palpating and visualizing the bisection of the calcaneus.

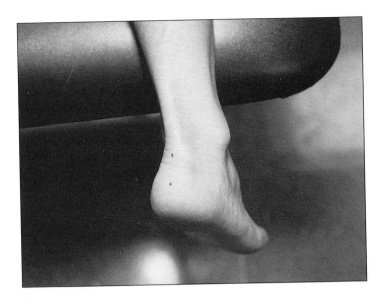

Figure 4.7   Placing two dots on the calcaneus that represent the line of bisection of the calcaneus.

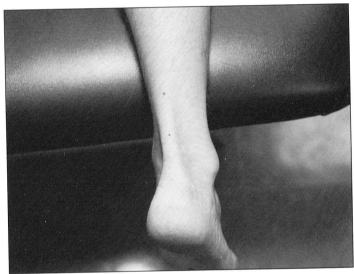

Figure 4.8   Dots on the lower one-third of lower leg representing the line of bisection.

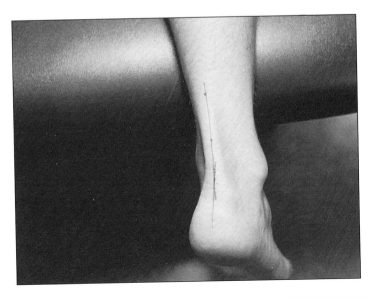

Figure 4.9   Draw the two lines of bisection.

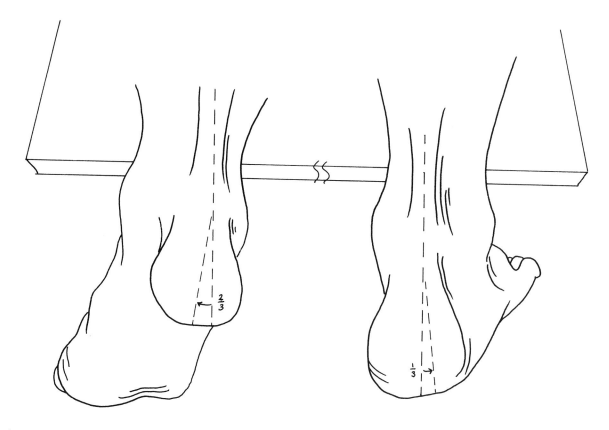

Figure 4.10 Two-thirds of subtalar motion should be inversion, one-third eversion.

Neutral position has also been defined with a forefoot component included, that is, with the subtalar joint in neutral and the midtarsal joint locked against the rearfoot. This is accomplished by applying a dorsiflexion force to the fourth and fifth metatarsals until resistance is felt. In this neutral position, the forefoot can be examined for structural or positional deformities. Some clinicians consider subtalar neutral to be the rearfoot component alone, while others consider it both the rearfoot and forefoot component of the exam. In this chapter, we will consider the subtalar joint and forefoot examinations separately.

There are two frequently used methods of determining neutral subtalar joint position. One is by palpation; the other is by calculations from the goniometric measurements. (Recent research regarding the reliability of each method is included in the following discussion of these techniques.) The clinician may choose to use either technique or a combination of the two for the clinical examination.

Palpation Method

Methods of placing the foot in neutral subtalar position have been described by a multitude of authors (D'Ambrosia & Douglas, 1982; Elveru, Rothstein, Lamb, & Riddle, 1988; James et al., 1978; McPoil & Brocato, 1985; Vogelbach & Combs, 1987). With the athlete in the prone position, palpate the medial and lateral aspects of the talus with your thumb and index finger. The medial aspect of the talus is found by palpating the talonavicular joint just anterior and inferior to the medial malleolus, as shown in Figure 4.11. The lateral head of the talus can be palpated just anterior of the sinus tarsi, as illustrated in Figure 4.12. Grasping the foot, invert and evert the ankle until the talus is felt equally on both sides so that the talus is congruent with the navicular (see Figure 4.13, a & b). The subtalar joint is now in neutral position via the palpation method (Figure 4.14).

The palpation method is probably the one most commonly used for determining neutral subtalar position. However, it is sometimes difficult for

Palpating to Determine Neutral Subtalar Joint Position

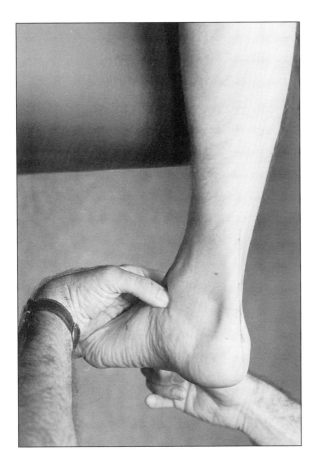

Figure 4.11 Palpating the medial head of the talus at the talonavicular joint.

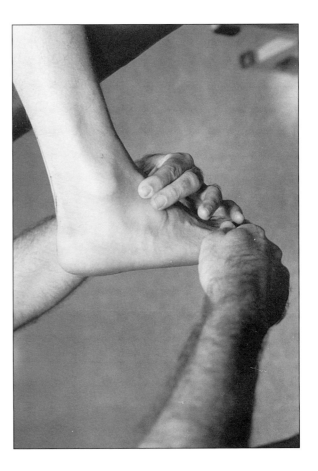

Figure 4.12 Palpating the lateral head of the talus.

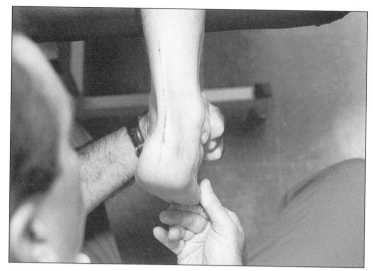

a

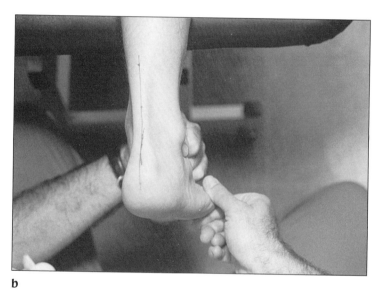

b

Figure 4.13 Invert (a) and evert (b) the calcaneus until the talus is felt equally on both sides.

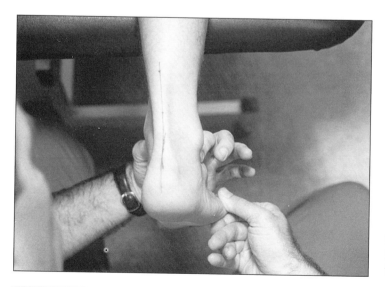

Figure 4.14 The foot is now in neutral subtalar joint position using the palpation technique.

clinicians to develop the feel for the technique. Due to its subjective nature, the reliability of this technique is frequently debated. In 1990, Smith-Oricchio and Harris reported moderate interrater reliability (ICC = 0.60) for the palpation method performed on subjects with recent ankle pathology.

Once neutral subtalar joint position has been determined by the palpation method, the rearfoot relationship can be determined. With the foot in neutral, the line of bisection on the calcaneus is compared visually to the line on the lower one-third of the leg. If the lines are parallel, the rearfoot is said to be neutral or zero degrees (see Figure 4.15). If the calcaneus is inverted in relation to the lower leg, the rearfoot is considered varus, as shown in Figure 4.16, and the angle should be measured with a goniometer or visually assessed for position and recorded on the evaluation sheet. The opposite deformity is a rearfoot valgus, with the calcaneus everted in relation to the lower leg's line of bisection, as illustrated in Figure 4.17. Again, the degree of deformity should be measured and recorded on the evaluation sheet. Be sure that the proper subtalar joint position is maintained during the measurement.

Goniometric Measurement Method

The goniometric method of determining neutral subtalar joint position uses the premise that the amount of inversion and eversion of the subtalar joint accounts for two-thirds and one-third, respectively, of the entire range of motion (Root et al., 1971). Thus the neutral position may be calculated from measurement of the passive range of motion of the calcaneus.

Measurement Procedure

With the patient in the prone position (as described above), measure the maximum amount of passive calcaneal inversion and eversion. To measure inversion, align the axis of the goniometer with the inferior edge of the lateral malleolus. Align the distal arm with the line of bisection through the calcaneus and align the proximal arm with the line bisecting the lower

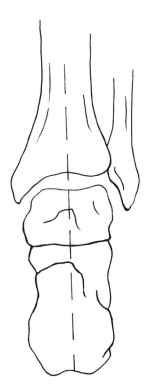

Figure 4.15 Neutral rearfoot position.

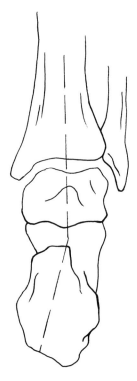

Figure 4.16 Rearfoot varus: the calcaneus is inverted in relation to the lower leg.

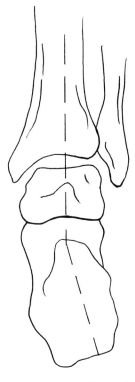

Figure 4.17 Rearfoot valgus: the calcaneus is everted in relation to the lower leg.

one-third of the lower leg. Grasp the calcaneus with thumb and index finger, forming a cup with the web space, and move the calcaneus to maximal inversion. Record the measurement (see Figure 4.18). Next measure maximal eversion and record the measurement, as shown in Figure 4.19.

Calculating Neutral Subtalar Joint Position From Goniometric Measurements

The neutral subtalar joint position (NSTJP) can be calculated by the following formula, adapted from the work of Root et al. (1971):

NSTJP = max. inversion + max. eversion / 3.

The result of this equation tells how far the calcaneus should be returned, measuring from the point of maximum eversion, to obtain the neutral subtalar joint position. As an example, suppose a clinician measures a maximum inversion of 20 degrees and maximum eversion of 10 degrees, making a sum of 30 degrees total range of movement (ROM). Dividing by 3, as prescribed by the formula, we obtain

NSTJP = (20 + 10) / 3 = 10 degrees.

Thus to position the subtalar joint at neutral, we would return the calcaneus 10 degrees from maximum eversion.

In this example, the inversion and eversion measurements tally exactly with the two-thirds to one-third ratio assumed in goniometric methodology. In most cases this model relationship is not present, but the same methodology is followed to determine neutral position regardless of the amount of inversion and eversion that is present. To take another example, suppose maximum inversion is 24 degrees and maximum eversion is 6 degrees. By the formula

NSTJP = (24 + 6) / 3 = 10 degrees,

total ROM is again 30, and dividing by 3 yields 10 degrees eversion from NSTJP. Therefore to place the subtalar joint in neutral we would move it 10 degrees from maximal eversion. In this example, the subtalar joint only has 6 degrees of eversion motion; therefore to place the joint in neutral we would have to move 4 additional degrees into inversion. Looking at one more example, let's assume 22 degrees maximum inversion, 5 degrees maximum eversion:

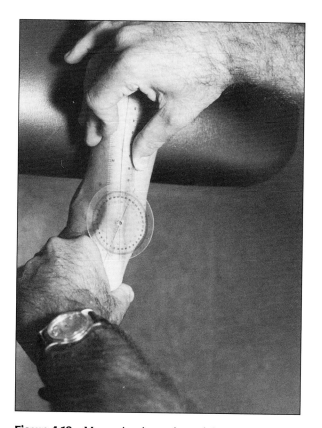

Figure 4.18 Measuring inversion of the calcaneus.

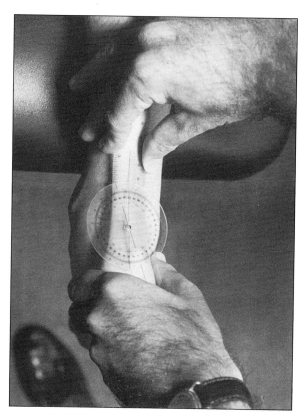

Figure 4.19 Measuring eversion of the calcaneus.

NSTJP = (22 + 5) / 3 = 9 degrees.

In this example, 9 degrees from maximal eversion would place the calcaneus in 4 degrees of inversion, which would be the neutral position of the subtalar joint in this patient.

In 1988, Elveru, Rothstein, and Lamb published research on the reliability of goniometric measurements in evaluation of the subtalar and ankle joints. The research was followed by a separate report addressing the issue from a clinical standpoint (Elveru, Rothstein, Lamb, & Riddle, 1988). The results showed intertester reliability coefficients of 0.32 for measurements of inversion unreferenced to neutral, 0.17 for eversion, and 0.25 for palpating subtalar joint neutral. When referenced to neutral subtalar joint position, these measurements had even lower intraclass coefficients. The authors recommend that measurements not be referenced from neutral subtalar joint position to improve their reliability. These papers address several points that have been debated by clinicians who use goniometric measurements in orthotic fabrication. The studies call into question the frequently used clinical criterion that inversion should account for two-thirds of the total range of motion, and eversion of the calcaneus should equal one-third. Smith-Oricchio and Harris (1990) report low intertester reliability coefficients for non-weightbearing calcaneal inversion and eversion measurements (0.42 and 0.25, respectively). Due to these low coefficient values, statistical analysis of determining neutral position by the calculation method was not performed.

Alternate Technique for Goniometric Measurements

Several reasons for inconsistent measurements of subtalar joint measurements have been suggested. They include lack of practice, inconsistent procedures, lack of consistent pressure on the calcaneus to achieve uniform end-feel, and difficulty in taking the measurements. Some clinicians find it difficult to hold the goniometer, maintain neutral subtalar joint position, and measure the foot and ankle simultaneously. An alternate technique is to hold the goniometer in one hand with both arms distal to the axis. Align one arm with the line of bisection of the lower leg and the other with the line through the calcaneus. Move the calcaneus into maximal inversion and eversion and record the appropriate measurements as shown in Figure 4.20, a & b. Dolan, Tonsoline, Bibi, and Reeds (1993) compared the one-handed or alternate technique to the traditional technique for measuring subtalar inversion and eversion by two experienced clinicians on both feet of 40 high school athletes. No significant differences were found between the traditional and alternate technique for the right foot, but there was a difference for the left foot (1.2 degrees). Interrater reliability coefficients of .50 and .82 were calculated for the right and left foot respectively using the traditional method. The alternate method yielded interrater values of .84 and .89. In addition, students who are learning gonimetric measurements of the subtalar joint subjectively comment that the one-handed method is simpler to perform.

These studies raise pertinent points regarding the reliability of measurements that many clinicians advocate as a critical portion of the biomechanical examination and eventual orthotic prescription. Clinicians who use these measurements must be aware of the possibility of error associated with them, as well as individual variations between patients from the 2:1 ratio of inversion to eversion in the subtalar joint. Standardization of procedures and practicing the techniques would appear to increase the reproducibility of the measurements.

Forefoot Evaluation

The next portion of the examination is the evaluation of the forefoot. Root et al. (1971) described the method of placing the subtalar joint in neutral position and placing the midtarsal joint in a pronated position to examine for forefoot deformities. First, place the subtalar joint in neutral position by palpation or calculation, according to the clinician's preference, and then grasp the fourth and fifth metatarsals and apply a dorsiflexion force until resistance is felt, thereby locking the midtarsal joint in a pronated position, as illustrated in Figure 4.21. The orientation of the forefoot will be assessed while the foot is held in this position. Figure 4.22 illustrates the three possible positions of the forefoot: neutral, varus, and valgus.

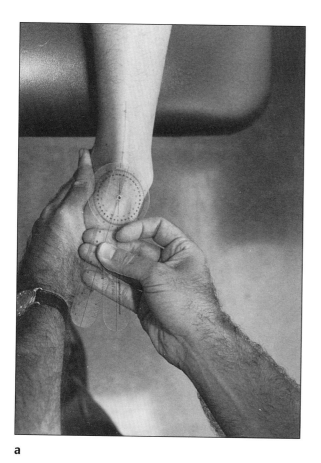
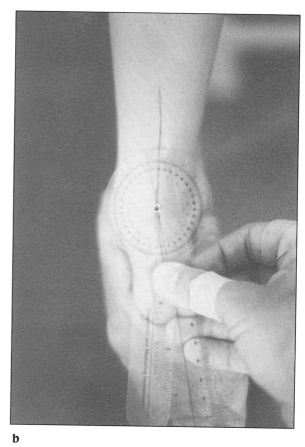

a   b

Figure 4.20   One-handed technique for measuring inversion (a) and eversion (b).

Neutral Forefoot

With the subtalar joint in neutral and the midtarsal joints pronated, the plane of the metatarsal heads should be perpendicular to the line of bisection of the calcaneus. Place one arm of the goniometer along the plantar aspect of the metatarsal heads and the other arm perpendicular to the orientation of the calcaneus while it is held in neutral position. In a neutral forefoot, the goniometer will read zero degrees.

Forefoot Varus

With forefoot varus, the forefoot is in a position of inversion when the subtalar joint is maintained in neutral and the midtarsal joints are fully pronated (Root et al., 1977). To measure the angle of forefoot varus, place one arm of the goniometer along the heads of the metatarsal with the axis lateral to the foot; the other

arm should be placed perpendicular to the calcaneal line of bisection, as shown in Figure 4.23. Circle the forefoot varus icon, and record the degrees of the measurement on the worksheet. Measurements of forefoot varus deformity averaged 8.4 degrees in a group of 52 subjects fitted for orthotic devices in a study by Donatelli, Hurlbert, Conaway, and St. Pierre (1988).

Forefoot Valgus

The opposite deformity, forefoot valgus, is the forefoot in a position of eversion with the subtalar joint maintained in neutral position and the midtarsal joint pronated (Root et al., 1977). To measure the angle of forefoot valgus, place one arm of the goniometer along the heads of the metatarsal with the axis medial to the foot; the other arm should be placed perpendicular to the calcaneal line of bisection with the subtalar joint maintained in neutral, as pictured in Figure 4.24.

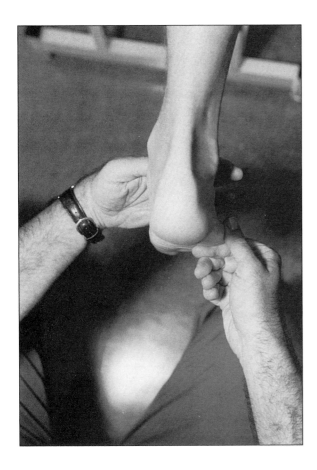

Figure 4.21   Place the foot in neutral subtalar joint position and apply a dorsiflexion force to the fourth and fifth metatarsals to assess for forefoot deformities.

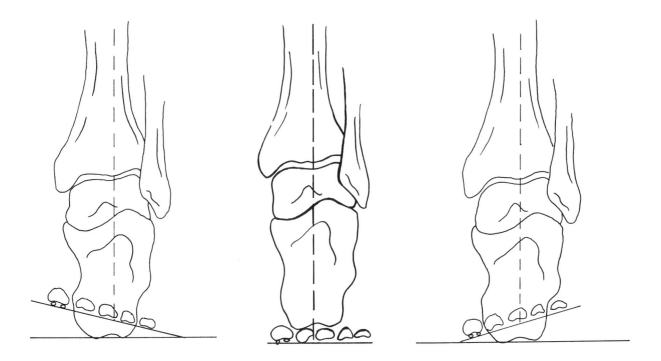

Figure 4.22   Forefoot varus, neutral, and valgus.

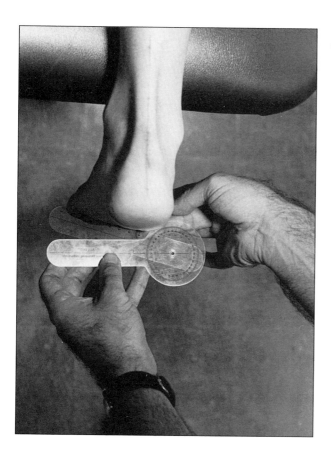

Figure 4.23 Measurement of forefoot varus: The forefoot is inverted in relation to the rearfoot in neutral subtalar joint position.

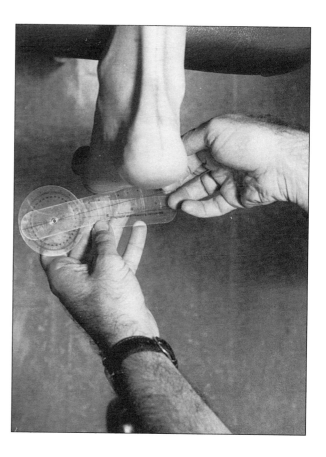

Figure 4.24 Measurement of forefoot valgus: The forefoot is everted in relation to the rearfoot in neutral subtalar joint position.

Examination of the First Ray

The first ray is formed by the functional unit of the first metatarsal and first cuneiform. Examination of the first ray is performed to determine (1) whether it is in dorsiflexed, plantar-flexed, or neutral position and (2) the range of motion in the joint. The patient can remain in the prone position; however, the authors prefer to place the patient in a supine position for this portion of the examination.

Position of the First Ray

Neutral position of the first ray has the first metatarsal in the same transverse plane as the central three metatarsal heads when they are maximally dorsiflexed (Root et al., 1977). With the patient supine, and the subtalar joint in neutral and the midtarsal joint pronated, visualize the position of the first metatarsal in relation to the four other metatarsal heads. With one thumb under the first metatarsophalangeal and the other thumb in line with the plane of the four lesser metatarsal heads, visualize the position of the metatarsal. If the thumbs lie in the same plane, the first ray is in normal position. If the thumb under the first metatarsal is dorsiflexed in reference to the four lesser metatarsals, the first ray is dorsiflexed. Accordingly, if the thumb under the first metatarsal is plantar-flexed in relation to the four lesser metatarsals, the first ray is considered plantar-flexed (Figure 4.25). Distinguishing between a plantar-flexed first ray and a forefoot valgus deformity can be difficult. A forefoot valgus is considered an osseous structural deformity while a plantar-flexed first ray is a positional deformity. Time should be taken to determine which of the two exist because the orthotic posting techniques for each condition are different.

Range of Motion of the First Ray

To determine the range of motion in the first ray, grasp the first metatarsal phalangeal joint between thumb and index finger, and move the joint into a dorsiflexed position and then into a plantar-flexed position, as shown in Figure 4.26. Root et al. (1977) state that the dorsiflexion and plantar flexion movements of the first ray should be equal, using the plane of the lesser metatarsal heads as

the reference point. Bordelon (1990) has indicated that 20 degrees of dorsiflexion and plantar flexion should be available at the joint. We do not take a goniometric measurement for this value; however, if you wish to, a text on podiatric goniometric values is suggested.

Dorsiflexion of the First Metatarsophalangeal Joint

The amount of dorsiflexion in the first metatarsophalangeal (MTP) joint is the last parameter evaluated on the first ray. The axis of the goniometer is placed at the metatarsophalangeal joint, and the arms are placed in line with the first metatarsal and first phalange, respectively, as shown in Figure 4.27a. Record the measurement on the worksheet. Root (1971) suggests that a minimum of 60 to 65 degrees of extension be present at the MTP joint for normal gait.

Ankle Joint Dorsiflexion

The ability of the ankle joint to dorsiflex a minimum of 10 degrees is necessary for normal gait. If dorsiflexion is not within normal limits, the foot and ankle complex may compensate abnormally, usually in the form of excessive pronation (Root et al., 1977). While the minimum 10 degrees of dorsiflexion is necessary for normal locomotion, it may be inadequate for running and jumping in athletic events.

With the patient in the prone position, align the arms of the goniometer with the fibula and the shaft of the fifth metatarsal. It is critical that the dorsiflexion measurements be taken with the foot in neutral subtalar joint position; therefore the lines of bisection on the lower leg and calcaneus should be observed. Allowing the foot to pronate during the dorsiflexion measurement will give an inaccurate value.

Two measurements are taken, one with the knee extended and the other with the knee flexed (Figures 4.28 and 4.29). The knee-extended measurement is more indicative of limitation of the gastrocnemius, while the knee-flexed measurement, when dorsiflexion is limited, indicates tightness of the soleus or significant joint pathology.

Figure 4.25   Positional assessment of the first ray: (a) normal, (b) dorsiflexed, and (c) plantar-flexed.

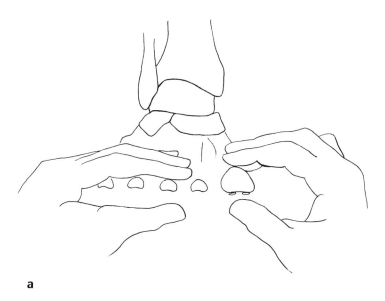

a

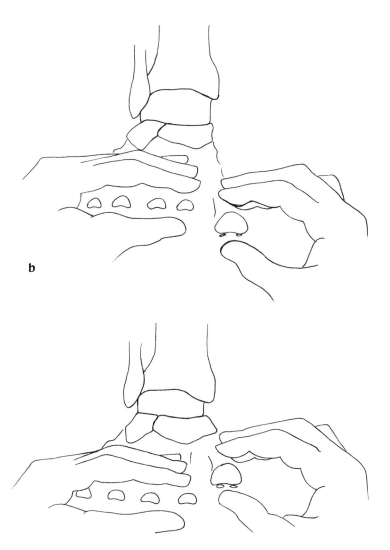

b

c

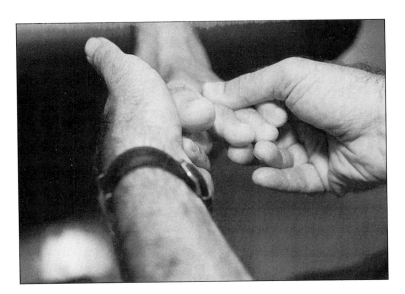

a

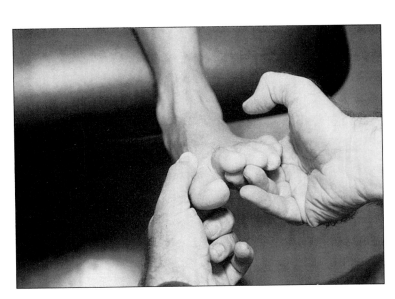

b

Figure 4.26   Determining range of motion in dorsiflexion (a) and plantar flexion (b) of the first ray.

Information derived from these measurements will guide the clinician in development of the total treatment plan, particularly in regard to stretching the appropriate structures of the lower leg and foot and ankle complex. The presence of ankle equinus is a critical factor in the decision-making process when considering orthotic management. Ankle joint equinus is defined as a lack of ankle joint dorsiflexion, most commonly attributed to limitation in the gastrocnemius and soleus muscle groups. The use of heel lifts to relieve stress on the gastrocnemius/soleus complex should be carefully considered by the clinician. Though effective for relieving symptoms, the injudicious use of a lift can cause additional functional shortening of the gastrocnemius/soleus unit

if an aggressive stretching program is not used in conjunction with the orthotic device. We feel that these patients should be treated with an aggressive stretching program of open and closed chain exercise. McPoil and Brocato (1985) consider a functional equinus of the ankle joint a contraindication to orthotic therapy.

Weightbearing Measurements

The next portion of the objective examination is to take a series of measurements in a weightbearing position. These measurements provide valuable information to the clinician about how the patient compensates for mechanical or positional

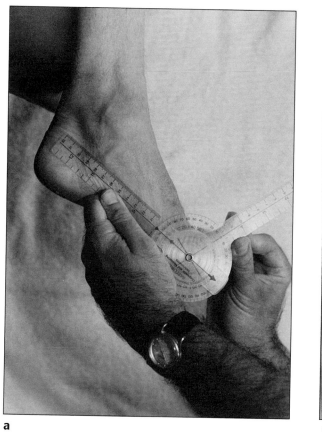

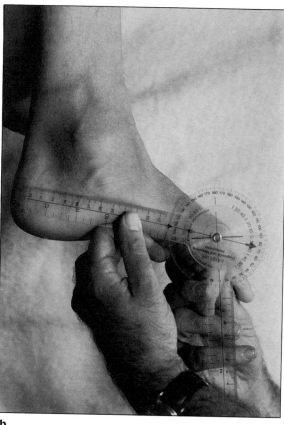

a

b

Figure 4.27 Measuring dorsiflexion (a) and plantar flexion (b) of the first metatarsophalangeal joint.

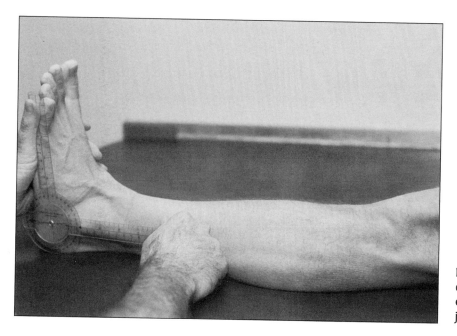

Figure 4.28 Measuring ankle dorsiflexion with the knee extended and the subtalar joint in neutral.

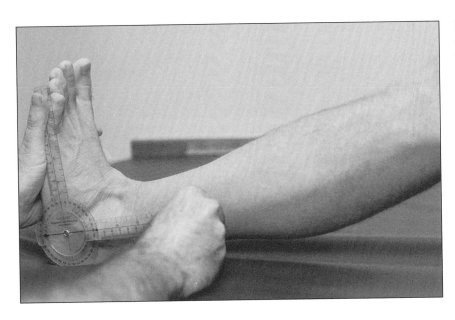

Figure 4.29 Measuring ankle dorsiflexion with the knee flexed and the subtalar joint in neutral.

deformities found in the non-weightbearing portion of the examination. Evaluative measurements and observations in the closed chain position should correlate to findings from the open chain or non-weightbearing examination.

Placement of the Foot in Neutral Subtalar Joint Position in Weightbearing

The following method for placing the subtalar joint in neutral is described by McPoil and Brocato (1985). With the patient standing on a firm surface, palpate the talus medially and laterally as previously described for the non-weightbearing position. Have the patient rotate the trunk to the left and right, causing an accompanying pronation and supination of the talus as the clinician palpates the structure. When the talus is felt equally on both sides and the talonavicular joint is congruent, the foot is considered neutral, as shown in Figure 4.30.

Measurement of Tibial Varum/Valgus

The alignment of the tibia in a weightbearing position affects the biomechanics of the foot and ankle. Therefore, tibial alignment will influence the eventual prescription for the orthotic device. Tibial varum is defined as the position in which the distal tibia is closer to the midline than the proximal portion of the tibia (McPoil & Brocato,

1985). This position is frequently referred to as bow-legged. The resulting inability of the medial portion of the foot to make full contact with the ground during the stance phase of gait can result in compensatory pronation (Root et al., 1977). Tibial valgus is the opposite deformity, defined as the position in which the distal tibia is lateral compared to the proximal tibia (see Figure 4.31).

The measurement is taken by aligning one arm of the goniometer with the lower leg bisection line and placing the other parallel to the floor, as shown in Figure 4.32. McPoil, Schuit, and Knecht (1988) compared three positions for measuring tibiofibular varum and determined that the resting calcaneal stance position was optimal for measurement.

Standing Calcaneal Inversion/ Eversion Measurement

This measurement is indicative of the amount of perpendicular calcaneal inversion or eversion present in a weightbearing position. Place one arm of the goniometer on the floor and align the other arm with the line of bisection on the calcaneus (Figure 4.33). When the calcaneus is everted, as would be expected in a pronated foot, this measurement indicates how far. It is important to keep in mind that the number of degrees that the calcaneus is everting is referenced not from the perpendicular position but rather from the neutral subtalar joint position of the calcaneus (Wooden, 1990). For example, if the neutral position of the

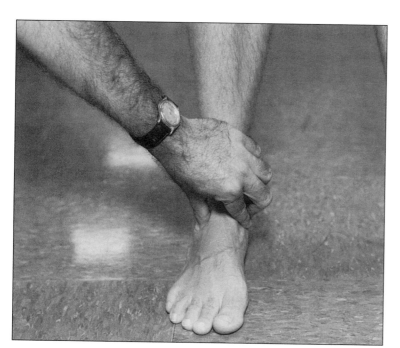

Figure 4.30 Placing the subtalar joint in neutral subtalar joint position in weightbearing.

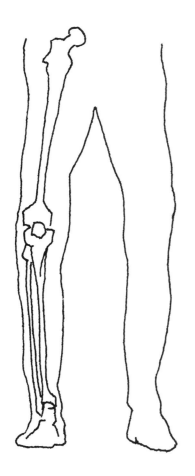

a   b

Figure 4.31 Tibial varum (a) and tibial valgus (b).

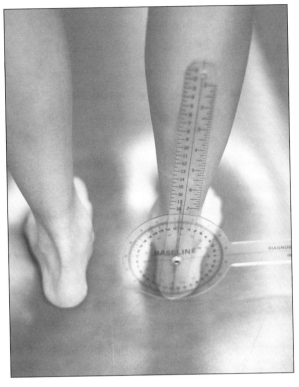

Figure 4.32 Measuring tibial position with a large plastic goniometer.

calcaneus is calculated as one degree of inversion, and the standing calcaneal measurement is 7 degrees of eversion, then the total amount of eversion is 8 degrees from neutral.

Lattanza, Gray, and Kantner (1988) conducted a study comparing the goniometric measurement of calcaneal eversion in a non-weightbearing position versus a weightbearing position. Weightbearing measurements of calcaneal eversion range of motion were significantly greater than non-weightbearing measurements by an average value of 37 percent. Smith-Oricchio and Harris (1990), examining interrater reliability coefficients for weightbearing measurements, reported interclass coefficients of 0.91 in bilateral stance and 0.75 in unilateral stance. An interesting aspect of this study was the measurement of calcaneal position in unilateral stance. Since the typical gait cycle is a unilateral event during the support phase, non-weightbearing calcaneal eversion would appear to be a clinically relevant measurement. However, they did not find any statistical difference between non-weightbearing calcaneal eversion measurements in bilateral stance versus unilateral stance.

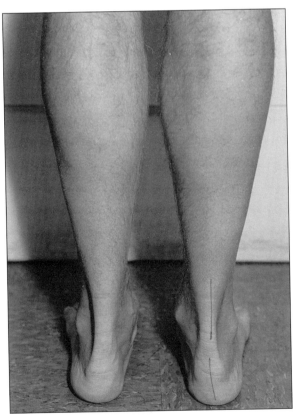

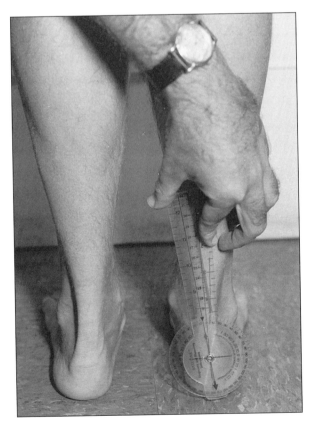

Figure 4.33 Calcaneal measurement to assess calcaneal inversion or eversion in weightbearing.

Navicular Differential

Navicular differential is a simple and relevant measurement of the dynamic changes that occur to the foot during weightbearing. When the foot goes into weightbearing, the navicular reacts to the changes in the subtalar joint as the foot pronates or supinates. When closed chain pronation occurs, the navicular moves downward as a result of the adduction and plantar flexion of the talus and eversion of the calcaneus, as illustrated in Figure 4.34. The amount of navicular drop is indicative of the amount of the pronation.

Have the patient sit in a chair with the knee bent to 90 degrees, and mark the navicular tuberosity with a pen (Figure 4.35). Placing the foot in neutral subtalar joint position, measure the distance from the mark to the floor (Figure 4.36). Have the patient stand up; measure the distance from the navicular to the floor (Figure 4.37). To determine navicular differential, subtract the semi-weightbearing measurement from the standing measurement. Brody (1982) considers normal values to be near 3/8 inch, or approximately 10 millimeters. A value over 5/8 inch, or 15 milli-meters, is considered excessive. Picciano, Rowlands, and Worrell (1993) examined intratester and intertester reliability of two inexperienced clinicians in measuring navicular drop. The intratester values were .61 and .79, with .57 recorded for the intertester values. They suggest that this measurement be practiced and not be used from one clinician to another due to low intertester reliability scores.

Q Angle

Q angle is a measurement of the alignment of the extensor mechanism of the knee. The axis of the goniometer is first aligned with the center of the patella. The distal arm is aligned with the tibial tuberosity and the proximal arm with the anterior superior iliac spine (Figure 4.38). Opinions vary as to Q angle values that contribute to patellar tracking injuries. Magee (1992) suggests that a Q angle of 13 to 18 degrees is normal. Females typically have a greater Q angle value than males. Our feeling is that a value in excess of 15 degrees in males or 20 degrees in females warrants clinical consideration.

Determining the Navicular Differential

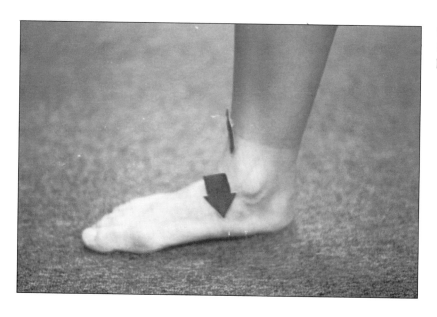

Figure 4.34 The navicular drops in a caudal direction during pronation.

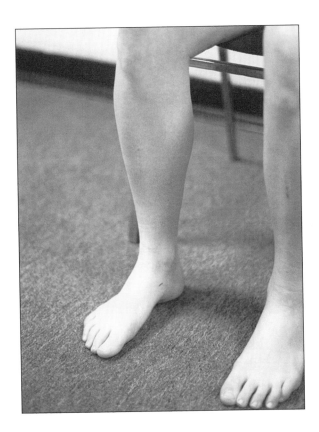

Figure 4.35 Mark the navicular tuberosity in a seated position.

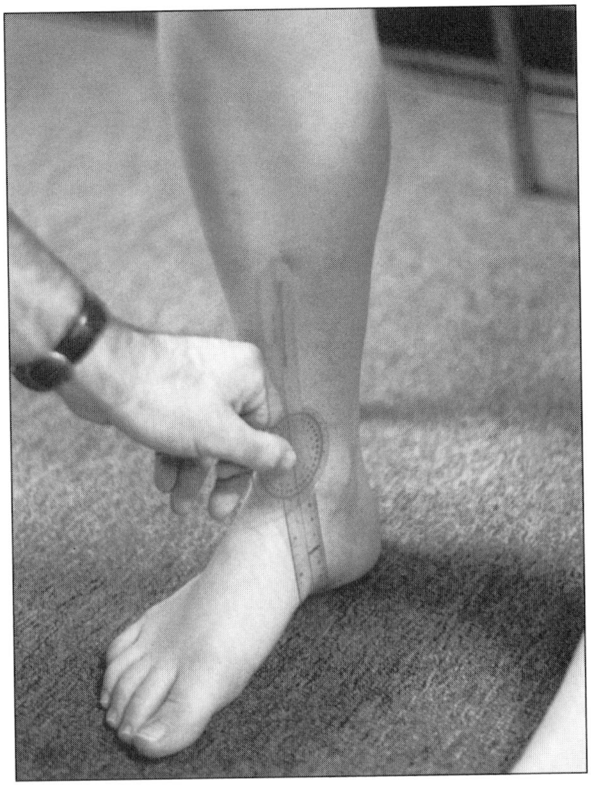

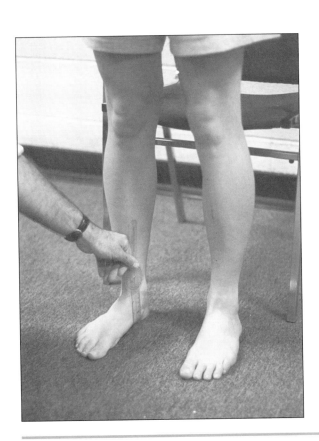

Figure 4.36 Measuring the distance from the navicular tuberosity to the floor, in seated position, to assess navicular differential.

Figure 4.37 Measuring the distance from the navicular tuberosity to the floor, in weightbearing position, to assess navicular differential.

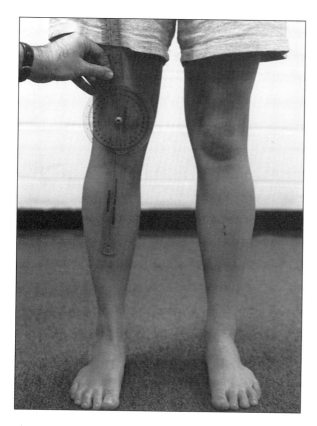

Figure 4.38 Measurement of Q angle.

A Angle

Arno (1990) introduced the measurement of the A angle as an indicator of patella alignment. A line is drawn through the longitudinal axis of the patella from the superior pole to the inferior pole. A second line is drawn from the tibial tubercle to the inferior pole of the patella. DiVeta and Vogelbach (1992) investigated the intratester and intertester reliability of A angle measurements. Their results indicated intratester reliability of .87 but intertester reliability of .59. In addition, comparing patients with patellofemoral signs to a control group, they found average A angle scores of 12.3 and 23.2 degrees for the control and symptomatic groups, respectively.

Gait Analysis

The final portion of the biomechanical examination is the dynamic evaluation of the patient's gait in walking and, especially when the patient is an athlete, running. It is important to remember that you will see variance in gait, especially when ana-

lyzing the gait of runners. An example is presented by Cavanagh (1987), who advocates the use of the term foot strike rather than heel strike because some runners never strike with their heels, as would be considered the norm. Mann and Hagy (1980) discusses gait cycle changes that occur in walking, running, and sprinting.

Gait analysis can be done on a flat surface or a treadmill, using direct observation or video camera or computer-based digitizer, depending on your time, budget, and expertise in operating the equipment. The clinicians seeking detailed knowledge of gait analysis are encouraged to consult these texts and publications: Cavanagh (1987); Donatelli (1987 & 1985); Inman, Rolston, and Todd (1981); Mann and Hagy (1980); Vogelbach (1988); Vogelbach and Combs (1987); Root et al. (1977); Tiberio (1987); Wooden (1990).

In addition to the lines of bisection on the lower leg and calcaneus, additional markings of important landmarks of the foot should be included for easier recognition of abnormal mechanics. These markings are the medial malleolus, navicular tubercle, and the medial aspect of the first MTP joint.

Stages of Gait

Gait can be described as a series of rotations occurring in the transverse plane that are transmitted through the ankle and subtalar joints, terminating with the bones of the foot (Mann & Hagy, 1980). The stance and swing phases are the major components of the gait cycle.

Stance Phase

The stance phase comprises approximately 60 percent of the gait cycle while the patient is walking. As the speed of ambulation increases from walking to running, stance decreases to 31 percent of the cycle. Stance phase drops to 22 percent of the gait cycle as the patient sprints (Mann & Hagy, 1980). This decrease in the stance phase may make it difficult for the clinician to determine abnormalities in the gait cycle during running or sprinting. However, with experience the clinician will begin to observe differences in gait that will be clinically relevant. The stance phase is broken down into three distinct sections: heel strike, midstance, and push-off.

Heel Strike

As the heel contacts the ground, it should be inverted, indicating that the subtalar joint is supinated (Figure 4.39). The supinated position provides a rigid lever for heel strike. The tibia is externally rotated, which can be verified by observing the line of bisection of the lower one-third of the lower leg.

Midstance

After heel strike, the foot must pronate to become a flexible unit to accommodate changes in the ground surface and to absorb the shock of gait. The foot moves into closed kinetic chain pronation by calcaneal eversion, plantar flexion and adduction of the talus, and eversion of the midtarsal joint. The clinician should see the calcaneus move into an everted position, as illustrated in Figure 4.40. At this point, the midtarsal joint becomes more parallel, which should be observed in the gait analysis as a dropping of the navicular (Figure 4.41). This pronation movement should be present for only the first 25 percent of the midstance phase. If the foot continues to pronate after this stage, the movement is considered ab-

normal. After 25 percent of midstance, the foot should begin to reverse toward supination to prepare for push-off.

Push-Off

In push-off, the foot continues to supinate to become a rigid lever for effective propulsion. The midtarsal joint moves from a pronated, or parallel, position to a supinated, or more oblique, axis. In this oblique position the stabilized midtarsal joint and supinated subtalar joint allow the foot to function as a rigid lever. This resupination will be observed as inversion of the calcaneus and an upward movement of the navicular (Figure 4.42). A rapid movement of the heel at push-off can indicate a limitation of the gastrocnemius/soleus complex (Vogelbach, 1988). If the foot remains pronated during any part of push-off, it is considered abnormal.

The rigidity of the foot is increased as the toes extend and weight is transferred from the lateral to the medial aspect of the foot. Toe extension should be observable at the marking of the first MTP joint. Extension of the toes tightens the plantar aponeurosis, which causes the medial longitudinal arch to tighten due to the windlass principle.

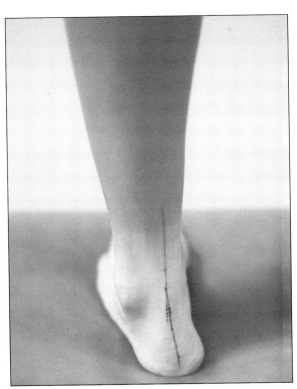

Figure 4.39 The calcaneus should be inverted at heel strike.

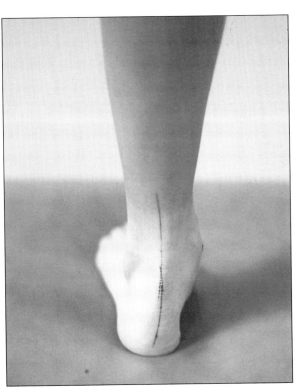

Figure 4.40 The calcaneus moves into an everted position as the foot pronates during early midstance.

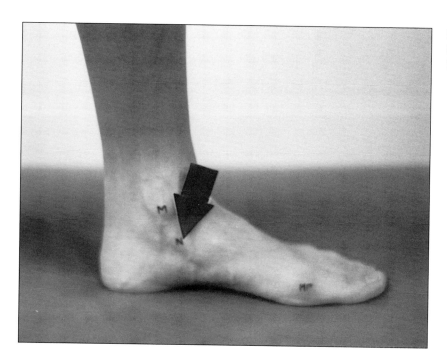

Figure 4.41 The navicular drops as the midtarsal joint becomes fully pronated during midstance.

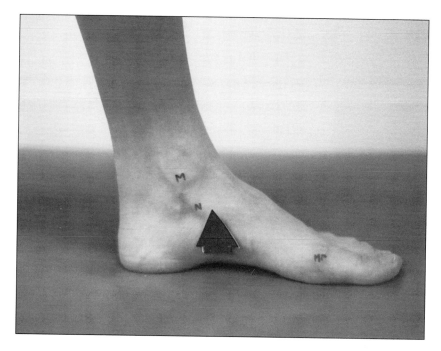

Figure 4.42 The navicular rises as the midtarsal joint axis becomes more oblique during supination.

If the foot does not supinate at the proper time in the gait cycle, external rotation of the tibia does not occur. This lack of external rotation of the tibia or prolonged internal rotation of the tibia can cause abnormal mechanics to more proximal structures of the lower kinetic chain.

Swing Phase

The swing phase accounts for approximately 40 percent of the gait cycle during walking. During swing, the lower kinetic chain prepares for the next heel strike.

Shoe Wear Pattern

The final portion of the gait analysis is an examination of the patient's shoes and athletic footwear. The wear patterns on the bottom of the shoe are indicative of where the forces of gait are being transmitted. In a normal wear pattern, the lateral portion of the heel should be worn, indicating the heel is supinated at heel strike. As the foot pronates and then supinates prior to push-off, the weight should transfer to the medial forefoot and show wear along the first metatarsal as it bears weight. Observation of the heel counter can indicate if the athlete displays abnormal pronation or supination (Figure 4.43). These variations in shoe pattern should correlate to what the clinician is observing during the dynamic gait analysis.

Figures 4.44 and 4.45 show two examples of abnormal shoe wear pattern.

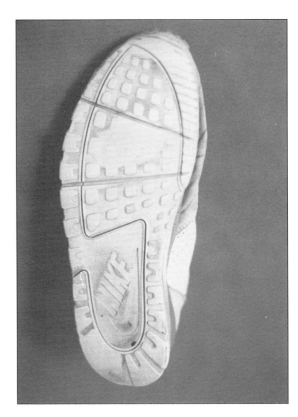

Figure 4.44 Shoe wear caused by fully compensated forefoot varus leading to abnormal pronation. Note the excessive wear pattern under the second and third metatarsal heads, due to the first metatarsal's hypermobility and inability to bear weight.

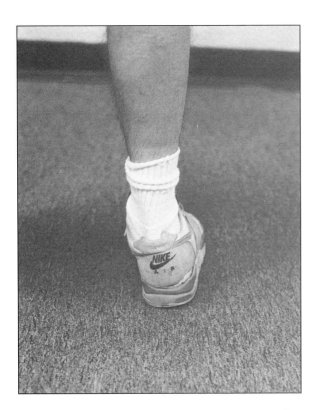

Figure 4.43 Deformed heel counter due to excessive pronation.

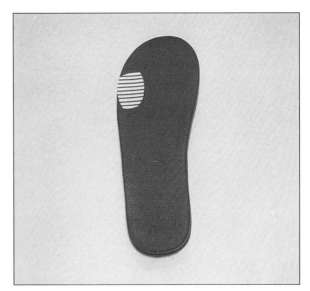

Figure 4.45 Model showing excessive wear on lateral forefoot caused by uncompensated forefoot varus.

Summary

This chapter introduced the biomechanical examination of the foot as a critical step in determining whether foot orthotics are indicated as part of the treatment plan. History, determining neutral subtalar joint position, open and closed chain measurements, and gait analysis have been discussed. Through research and clinical trial and error, each clinician will determine the preferred examination techniques suitable to their clinical setting and professional choices.

References

Arno, S. (1990). The A angle: A quantitative measurement of patella alignment and realignment. *The Journal of Orthopaedic and Sports Physical Therapy, 12*, 237–242.

Bordelon, M.L. (1990). Clinical assessment of the foot. In R. Donatelli, (Ed.), *The biomechanics of the foot and ankle* (pp. 85–97). Philadelphia: Davis.

Brody, D.M. (1982). Techniques in evaluation and treatment of the injured runner. *Orthopedic Clinics of North America, 13*, 541–558.

Cavanagh, P.R. (1987). The biomechanics of lower extremity action in distance running. *Foot and Ankle, 7*, 197–217.

D'Ambrosia, R.D., & Douglas, C.P. (1982). Orthotics. In R.D. D'Ambrosia & D. Drez (Eds.), *Prevention and treatment of running injuries* (pp. 155–164). Thorofare, NJ: Slack.

DiVeta, J.A., & Vogelbach, W.D. (1992). The clinical efficacy of the A-angle in measuring patellar alignment. *The Journal of Orthopaedic and Sports Physical Therapy, 16*, 136–139.

Dolan, M.G. (1983). *The effect of a semi-rigid orthotic on pain from shinsplints.* Unpublished master's thesis, University of North Carolina at Chapel Hill.

Dolan, M.G., Tonsoline, P.A., Bibi, K.W., & Reeds, G.K. (1993). Validity and reliability of an alternate method of measuring subtalar joint inversion and eversion. *Proceedings of 1993 National Athletic Trainers Association Convention, 28*(2), 154.

Donatelli, R. (1985). Normal biomechanics of the foot and ankle. *The Journal of Orthopaedic and Sports Physical Therapy, 7*, 91–95.

Donatelli, R.A. (1987). Abnormal biomechanics of the foot and ankle. *The Journal of Orthopaedic and Sports Physical Therapy, 9*, 11–16.

Donatelli, R., Hurlbert, C., Conaway, D., & St. Pierre, R. (1988). Biomechanical foot orthotics: A retrospective study. *The Journal of Orthopaedic and Sports Physical Therapy, 10*, 205–212.

Elveru, R.A., Rothstein, J.M., & Lamb, R.L. (1988). Goniometric reliability in a clinical setting: Subtalar and ankle joint measurements. *Physical Therapy, 68*, 672–677.

Elveru, R.A., Rothstein, J.M., Lamb, R.L., & Riddle, D.L. (1988). Methods for taking subtalar joint measurements: A clinical report. *Physical Therapy, 68*, 678–682.

Greenfield, B. (1990). Evaluation of overuse syndromes. In R. Donatelli (Ed.), *The biomechanics of the foot and ankle* (pp. 153–177). Philadelphia: Davis.

Inman, V.T., Rolston, H.J., & Todd, F. (1981). *Human walking.* Baltimore: Williams & Wilkins.

James, S.L., Bates, B.T., & Osternig, L.R. (1978). Injuries to runners. *The American Journal of Sports Medicine, 6*, 40–50.

Lattanza, L., Gray, G.W., & Kantner, R.M. (1988). Closed versus open kinematic chain measurements of subtalar joint eversion: Implications for clinical practice. *The Journal of Orthopaedic and Sports Physical Therapy, 9*, 310–314.

Magee, D.J. (1992). *Orthopedic physical assessment.* Philadelphia: Saunders.

Mann, R.A., & Hagy, J. (1980). Biomechanics of walking, running, and sprinting. *The American Journal of Sports Medicine, 8*, 345–350.

McPoil, T.G., & Brocato, R.S. (1985). The foot and ankle: Biomechanical evaluation and treatment. In J.A. Gould & G.J. Davies (Eds.), *Orthopaedic and sports physical therapy* (Vol. 2, pp. 313–341). St. Louis: Mosby.

McPoil, T.G., Schuit, D., & Knecht, H.G. (1988). A comparison of three positions used to evaluate tibial varum. *Journal of the American Podiatric Medical Association, 78*, 22–28.

Picciano, A.M., Rowlands, M.S., & Worrell, T. (1993). Reliability of open and closed kinetic chain subtalar joint neutral positions and navicular drop test. *The Journal of Orthopaedic and Sports Physical Therapy, 18*(4), 553–558.

Root, M.L., Orien, W.P., & Weed, J.H. (1977). *Clinical biomechanics: Vol. II. Normal and abnormal function of the foot.* Los Angeles: Clinical Biomechanics.

Root, M.L., Orien, W.P., Weed, J.H., & Hughes, R.J. (1971). *Clinical biomechanics: Vol. I. Biomechanical examination of the foot.* Los Angeles: Clinical Biomechanics.

Smith-Oricchio, K., & Harris, B.A. (1990). Interrater reliability of subtalar neutral, calcaneal inversion and eversion. *The Journal of Orthopaedic and Sports Physical Therapy, 12*, 10–15.

Tiberio, D. (1987). The effect of excessive subtalar joint pronation on patellofemoral mechanics: A theoretical model. *The Journal of Orthopaedic and Sports Physical Therapy, 9*, 160–165.

Vogelbach, W.D. (1988). *The lower kinetic chain: Foundation for normal and abnormal function.* Morgantown, WV: Biomechanics.

Vogelbach, W.D., & Combs, L.C. (1987). A biomechanical approach to the management of chronic lower extremity pathologies as they relate to excessive pronation. *Athletic Training, 22*, 6–16.

Wooden, M. (1990). Biomechanical evaluation for functional orthotics. In R. Donatelli (Ed.), *The biomechanics of the foot and ankle* (pp. 131–147). Philadelphia: Davis.

5

Casting and Molds

The preceding chapter discussed and illustrated the procedures for performing a clinical examination to determine the necessity of orthotic therapy. This chapter discusses the methods of casting the foot in neutral subtalar joint position for the fabrication of rigid or semirigid orthotic therapy as part of the patient's overall treatment plan.

Making a Negative Cast

The purpose of casting the foot is to capture the neutral subtalar joint position, from which an orthotic device can eventually be produced. The technique has been described by a multitude of authors: D'Ambrosia (1985), Donatelli and Wooden (1990), McPoil and Brocato (1985), and Torg (1982). The cast is made in a non-weightbearing position with the patient either prone or supine, depending on the preference of the clinician.

Materials Needed

The following materials are needed to make a negative cast (see Figure 5.1):

- Two 5 × 30 inch (13 × 75 cm) fast-setting plaster splints, folded in half
- Basin of warm water
- Towels for floor and table
- Rubber gloves (optional)
- Scissors

Procedures

The patient is placed in the same position as for the biomechanical examination (Figure 5.2). In-struct the patient to relax the lower leg and ankle to ensure that the muscles are not contracting, which could result in an incorrect casting position. McPoil and Brocato (1985) cite the possibility of the anterior tibialis contracting during the casting procedure, yielding a false forefoot varus deformity in the cast.

After placing the first double-folded splint in the basin of water, remove excess water from the splint by squeezing it over the basin. Hold the splint in one hand above the basin, and with the thumb and index finger of the opposite hand smooth the splint of any wrinkles (Figure 5.3). This smoothing will also "cream" the splint by mixing the plaster with the bandage material, making it easier to work with and producing a smoother cast. Fold approximately 1/8 inch (3 mm) over the top edge of the splint; this fold will make it easier to remove the cast when it hardens (Figure 5.4). The first splint is placed posteriorly around the heel and extended to the metatarsal heads (Figure 5.5). The second splint is reversed, starting from the anterior portion of the toes and extending posterior to the heel (Figure 5.6). Smooth the splints with your hands to remove any ridges or creases in the cast.

At this point place the foot in neutral position. If using the palpation method, invert and evert the foot until the talus is felt evenly on both sides and is congruous with the navicular; grasp the fourth and fifth metatarsals and lock the midtarsal joints by applying a dorsiflexion force until resistance is felt. This procedure ensures that the midtarsal joints are fully pronated (Figure 5.7). If you use the goniometric method, place the subtalar joint in neutral as previously calculated and then pronate the midtarsal joints, as just described for the palpation method.

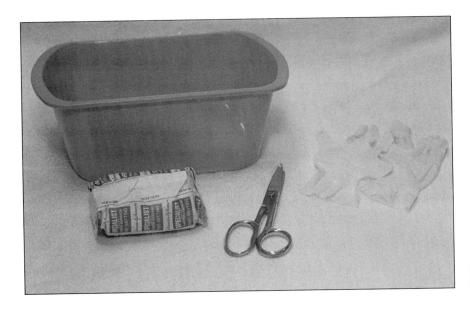

Figure 5.1   Materials needed to make a negative cast.

Casting

Figure 5.2   Patient positioning for making a cast with the foot in neutral subtalar joint position.

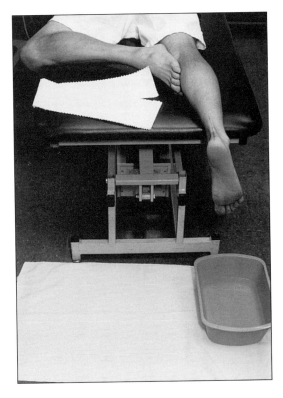

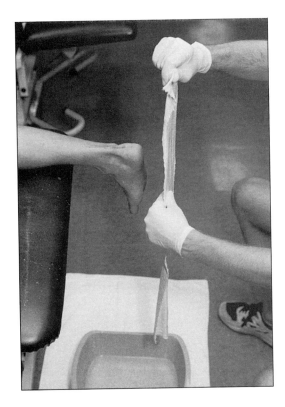

Figure 5.3   Smoothing and creaming the splints before application.

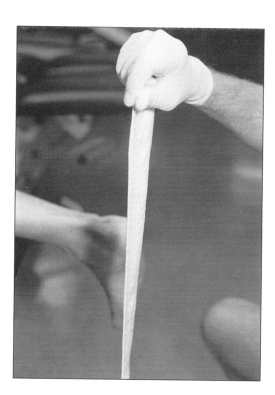

Figure 5.4 Fold the top edge of the splints approximately 3 millimeters (1/8 inch) to make them easier to remove when dry.

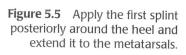

Figure 5.5 Apply the first splint posteriorly around the heel and extend it to the metatarsals.

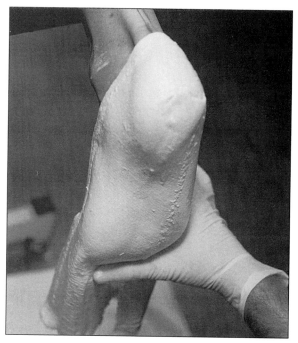

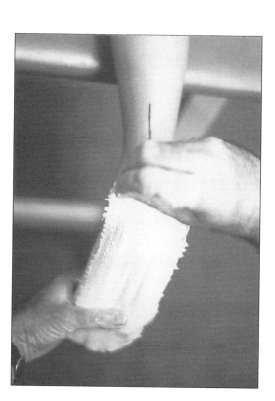

Figure 5.6 Apply the second splint from the anterior surface of the toe and extend it posteriorly.

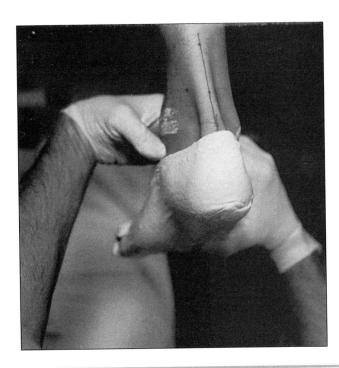

Figure 5.7 Place the foot in neutral subtalar joint position, and apply pressure at the fourth and fifth metatarsals to pronate the midtarsal joint. Allow the cast to harden while maintaining this position.

The cast can become misshaped when you are applying this dorsiflexion force. Some clinicians feel that excess dorsiflexion is a significant problem that can result in incorrect representation of the forefoot alignment and thus an incorrectly posted orthotic device. Donatelli and Wooden (1990) recommend applying a downward distraction on the fifth toe to prevent misshaping the cast. Philips (1990) suggests using a folded gauze bandage to act as a cushion to absorb the pressure on the fourth and fifth metatarsal heads. Colonna (1989) suggests pressing out the defect from the inside of the cast.

Maintain the neutral subtalar joint position until the cast hardens. At this point carefully remove the cast and allow to dry (Figure 5.8). The cast should represent the deformity in a neutral nonweightbearing position in relation to the rearfoot and forefoot alignment.

At this point the clinician may decide to send the cast to any of a wide variety of companies that will use the negative cast to fabricate a positive mold and then an orthotic. The clinician will have to fill out some type of shipping and instruction form for the company. This will usually include

- the type of orthotic device (rigid, semirigid, soft);
- the length of orthotic;
- the type of shoe the patient will wear with the orthotic;
- special adaptations to the orthotic: metatarsal lifts, relief areas, heel lifts, etc.; and
- posting instructions. Either you provide the types and angles for the forefoot and rearfoot, or you allow the lab to make that determination based on the positive molds that will be produced from your negative cast.

Supine Technique

Depending on the clinician's preference, the patient can be placed in a supine position for the casting, as described by Burns (1977) and shown in Figure 5.9. The same procedures as in the prone technique are employed for placing the subtalar joint and forefoot into neutral position.

Foam Impression Trays

Another method of obtaining an impression of the foot is using a foam impression box. In this method the patient is seated with hip and knee joint at 90 degrees. The clinician then presses the entire foot to the bottom of the tray (Figure 5.10). Other methods include placing and maintaining the subtalar joint in neutral while placing the foot into the foam box. If you have used a technique that is different

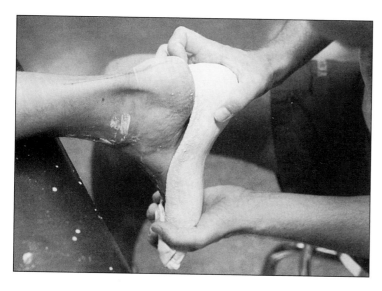

Figure 5.8 Remove the cast after it has dried.

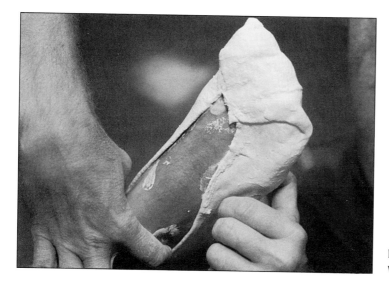

Figure 5.9 Making a negative cast with the patient supine.

from the manufacturer's suggestion, it is important to specify this to insure an acceptable orthotic device. The box is then packaged and shipped to the manufacturer for orthotic fabrication.

Comparing Impression Techniques

In a study comparing cast impression techniques, McPoil, Schuit, and Knecht (1989) considered prone non-weightbearing, supine non-weightbearing, and semi-weightbearing modes. Their data revealed that the two non-weightbearing techniques were reproducible, but the semi-weightbearing technique was subject to significant differences in goniometric measurements of the forefoot and rearfoot. The authors attributed these differences to the clinicians' not being able to load the midtarsal joints by applying dorsiflexion pressure to the fourth and fifth metatarsals when the patient is in the semi-weightbearing posture. Valmassey (1979) found similar results when using a semi-weightbearing technique. It should be noted that the foam technique also excludes the clinician from pressing on the midtarsal joints, which may explain why it is sometimes difficult to capture sagittal plane deformities with foam impression trays. This can be corrected by adding specific posting instructions to the orthotic prescription sent to the manufacturer. Regardless of the technique that you adopt, the key component is consistent reproducibility in your casting technique.

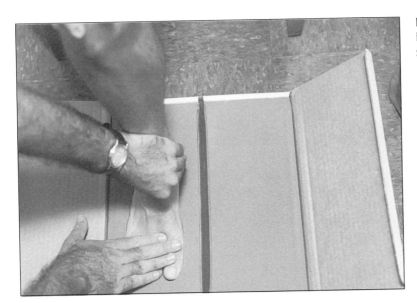

Figure 5.10 Use of a foam impression tray to capture neutral subtalar joint position.

a

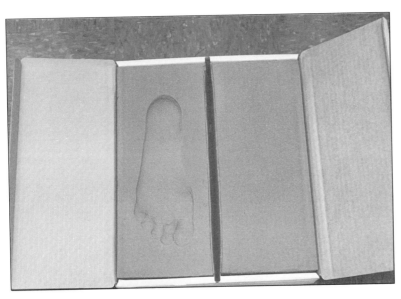

b

Making a Positive Mold

Once the negative cast has dried completely, a positive mold can be made from the cast. A mixture of plaster is poured into the negative slipper cast. After the positive has dried, the negative is torn from the positive mold. From the positive mold an orthotic device can be fabricated in a variety of ways. Clinicians may choose to make their own orthotics, which will require additional time, materials, and equipment. For readers who desire a more detailed description of making a positive mold, several texts and articles are listed in the references at the end of the chapter.

Materials Needed

The following materials are needed to make a positive mold:

- Plaster of Paris powder
- Cast separation material
- Water
- Rubber mixing bowl
- Spatula

Procedures

First, check the negative cast for cracks and ensure that it is deep enough to accept the liquid plaster. Philips (1990) recommends a minimum depth of 1/4 inch (6 mm) (Figure 5.11). If the cast is too shallow, the positive mold will be too shallow as well. A shallow mold can fracture when the thermoplastic material is applied, especially if a vacuum or hand press is used to form the orthotic on the mold. If the cast is too shallow, add another layer of plaster splints around the top border. Some type of cast-separating medium is poured and spread into the negative cast to allow easier separation of the dried positive mold from the negative cast. Sodium-alginate is one of the recommended cast separating substances, but inexpensive alternatives such as dishwashing detergent or foot and body powder produce ex-

cellent results. Coat the entire cast with the cast separating medium; then remove any excess material from the cast.

Mix approximately two pounds of plaster powder with warm water in a rubber bowl—Philips (1990) recommends one liter of water with 1.8 kilograms of plaster powder—until the mix is smooth and creamy. Pour a small amount of the plaster mixture into the negative cast, enough to line the entire cast. Slowly pour the remaining mixture into the cast until it is full. Gently tap the cast to eliminate as many air bubbles as possible. Allow at least 60 minutes for the mold to set. Remove the negative cast from the positive mold and continue with your orthotic prescription (Figure 5.12).

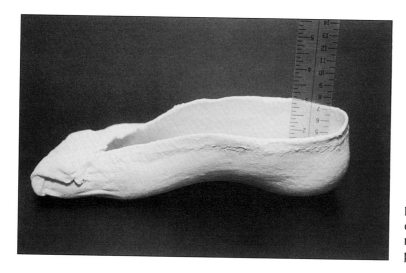

Figure 5.11 Check the negative cast for cracks. It must have a depth of 6 millimeters (1/4 inch) to accept the liquid plaster of Paris.

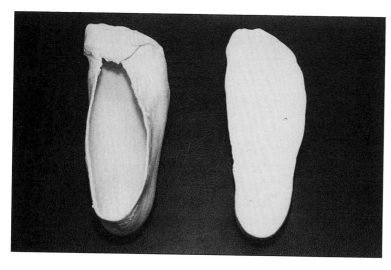

Figure 5.12 Separate the positive mold from the cast.

Summary

This chapter describes casting techniques for capturing neutral subtalar joint and foot position. These include non-weightbearing, weightbearing, and foam impression tray techniques. If the clinician wants a semirigid or rigid orthotic device, he or she can send the negative cast out to a variety of orthotic manufacturers. Though it is time consuming and requires specialized training, some clinicians create a positive mold and fabricate semirigid or rigid devices in their own clinical settings.

References

Burns, M.J. (1977). Non-weightbearing cast impressions for the construction of orthotic devices. *The Journal of the American Podiatry Association*, **67**, 790–794.

Colonna, P. (1989). Fabrication of a custom molded orthotic using an intrinsic posting technique for a forefoot varus deformity. *Physical Therapy Forum*, **8**, 6–7.

D'Ambrosia, R.D. (1985). Orthotic devices in running injuries. *Clinics in Sports Medicine*, **4**, 611–618.

Donatelli, R., & Wooden, M. (1990). Biomechanical orthotics. In R. Donatelli (Ed.), *The biomechanics of the foot and ankle* (pp. 193–216). Philadelphia: Davis.

McPoil, T.G., & Brocato, R.S. (1985). The foot and ankle: Biomechanical evaluation and treatment. In J.A. Gould & G.J. Davies (Eds.), *Orthopaedic and sports physical therapy* (Vol. 2, pp. 313–341). St. Louis: Mosby.

McPoil, T.G., Schuit, D., & Knecht, H.G. (1989). Comparison of three methods used to obtain a neutral plaster foot impression. *Physical Therapy*, **69**, 448–452.

Philips, J.W. (1990). *The functional foot orthosis*. New York: Churchill Livingstone.

Torg, J.S. (1982). Athletic footwear and orthotic appliances. *Clinics in Sports Medicine*, **1**, 157–175.

Valmassey, R.L. (1979). Advantages and disadvantages of various casting techniques. *Journal of the American Podiatric Association*, **69**, 707–712.

Equipment and Materials

6

There are probably as many ways to make orthotics as there are people making them. Everyone has favorite materials and techniques. This chapter will review many of the materials and pieces of equipment used in the fabrication of different types of orthotics.

Terminology

To understand better the characteristics that determine the effectiveness of an orthotic material, it is essential to define certain terms. These terms describe the properties that may be compared when choosing a material with which to work.

Several principles define the physical and mechanical properties of a material. Stress is the amount of force applied over a given area, expressed mathematically as force/area. There are three types of stress:

- Tensile stress is directed outward from the surface.

- Compressive stress is directed perpendicular to the surface.

- Shear stress is directed parallel to the surface.

Strain is the change per unit of length in response to stress. There are three types of stress-strain relationships (Murphy & Burnstein, 1975; Rome, 1991):

- Tensile, resulting in deformation by extension

- Compressive, resulting in deformation of thickness

- Shearing, resulting in deformation at right angles to the stress plane

Compression set is the amount of contraction of a material after it has been compressed for a certain compression strain or a given time. Compression set is given as a percentage either of the original dimension or of the total contraction. Campbell, Newell, and McLure (1982) tested 31 materials for compression in order to determine the suitability of the materials as shoe insoles. The researchers classified the materials as very stiff, moderately deformable, or very deformable. The ideal insole material was found to be one that deformed throughout the load but accommodated bony prominences so as to transfer some of the load to other regions. The very deformable materials reached complete compression or "bottomed out" quickly under relatively low stress. The very stiff materials deformed little, so there was no distribution of stress. The moderately deformable materials demonstrated the ideal qualities better than the other two types, deforming under stress but also transferring some of the pressure from bony prominences of the foot to adjacent structures.

Hardness is a measure of the resistance of a material to permanent distortion by indentation or scratching. Hardness is calculated by the ball indentation test. The size of the permanent impression left by a ball under a certain load is called the ball indentation hardness (Rome, 1990).

Resilience is the ability of a material to recover after compression. Resilience also represents the ability of a material to absorb energy (Gere & Timoshenko, 1984). Density, or the mass per unit of volume, correlates inversely with resilience. It is often used to compare the physical attributes of samples within a test group, to ensure their uniformity (Rome, 1991).

Materials

In the early years of orthotic usage, rubber, cork, and leather were predominant materials of manufacture (Campbell, Newell, & McLure, 1982). As usage increased with the popularity of running during the 1970s and 1980s, new materials were introduced, which led to lighter and more durable orthotics. Plastic synthetics have many of the qualities that are ideal for orthotics (Olson, 1988; Rome, 1990). The introduction of thermoplastics in the early 1970s brought on tremendous advances in design, versatility, and application. Thermoplastic materials are hypoallergenic, moisture- and bacteria-resistant, and heat moldable (White, 1992). Three types of plastics are commonly used in orthotics (Peppard & O'Donnell, 1983).

- Thermoforming plastics are formed, and may later be re-formed, by heat.
- Thermosetting plastics, made of cross-linked molecules, are difficult to re-form.
- Thermoplastics are rigid when cool but may be re-formed with heat. Thermoplastic foams are made by injection of gases at high temperature to change the density of the material.

As we have seen in earlier chapters, orthotics are often classified as soft, semirigid, or rigid, according to the material used in manufacture (Schwartz, 1991). The two main categories of orthotics are

- accommodative, cushioning the foot and relieving pressure in certain areas, and
- corrective, repositioning or supporting the foot in an ideal position.

With the advent of materials such as plastics, these categories of orthotics are not as clearly delineated as they once were. Certain materials or combinations of materials may belong to several categories or types of orthotics.

Soft Materials

Soft materials are used to cushion the foot and selectively reduce pressure on sensitive areas. Studies have shown that soft insoles reduce shock during walking or running. Early usage was for arthritis, diabetes, or leprosy (Enna, Brand, Reed, & Welch, 1976; Gould, 1982; Hertzman, 1973; Schwartz, 1991). Because soft materials are generally less durable, they tend to be thicker and so require a deeper shoe or more grinding. Often, a soft orthotic is prescribed as a temporary device to determine if an orthotic will be effective. If the soft, easy-to-manufacture orthotic proves effective, then a more rigid orthotic may be fabricated.

The most commonly used soft material today is Plastazote (Campbell, Newell, & McLure, 1982; Cracchiolo, 1982; Glass, Karno, Sella, & Zeleznik, 1982; Holmes, 1980). Plastazote is a cross-linked closed-cell polyethylene thermoplastic that has been in use as an orthotic material since 1969 (Schwartz, 1991). Thermoplastic means Plastazote will soften every time it is heated. It is water- and solvent-resistant. Holmes states that one of the few disadvantages to Plastazote is that, as a thermoplastic, it retains heat from the foot and may cause the foot to be hotter than otherwise and sweaty. For patients with a circulatory deficiency of the foot, the increased temperature may actually be an advantage. Plastazote comes in grades of firmness: grade 1 is medium, grade 2 is firm, and grade 3 is very firm or rigid. Firmer grades of Plastazote do not compress, or bottom out, as soon as less firm grades, but they also do not cushion as well. Material density ranges from 3 to 12 pounds per cubic foot. It may be fashioned into an orthotic insole or as a sandal with straps. Plastazote is heat malleable and autoadherent at approximately 240 °F (115 °C). From this temperature, it takes less than one minute to heat Plastazote to molding temperature. Plastazote is available in thicknesses ranging from 1/16 inch to one inch (Figure 6.1).

Aliplast 4E is another cross-linked closed-cell polyethylene foam that is considered a soft material. Five types of Aliplast vary in stiffness and firmness, with available densities ranging from 2 pounds per cubic foot for Aliplast 2E to 12 pounds per cubic foot for Aliplast 10. Grade 1 (soft) polyethylene foams like Aliplast 4E and Plastazote have compression sets of about 30 percent (Schwartz, 1991). Aliplast is autoadherable at approximately

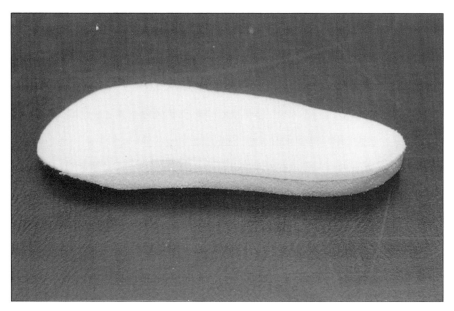

Figure 6.1 Soft Plastazote orthotic.

250 to 325 °F (120 to 160 °C), depending on the density, or grade, being heated. Its ability to adhere to other materials such as Plastazote at moderate temperatures can be advantageous in fashioning an orthotic. Aliplast bonds to polyethylene or polypropylene with strength that exceeds the foam itself. Because it is smoother in texture than Plastazote, Aliplast is often used as the liner material for an orthotic (Showers & Strunck, 1985). Aliplast will shrink along the length of the grain with heating, but the width of the material stays the same.

Pelite is a lightweight sponge foam polypropylene. It may be perforated or nonperforated. Perforated materials allow the passage of air to the tissues below, thereby reducing heat retention. Pelite becomes malleable at 265 °F (130 °C).

Polyurethane foam is another type of material that is growing in popularity for use in soft orthotics. The polyurethane is combined with a blowing agent to create a series of open-celled tunnels, which allow perspiration and heat to be dissipated from the foot. This material, available in sheets of various thicknesses, is used mainly in pressure absorbing orthotics. Patient Protective Technology (PPT) is one of the most popular trade names for this material.

Semirigid Materials

Semirigid orthotics are made of slightly firmer materials and incorporate posting techniques (Subotnick, 1975). Most semirigid orthotics are made of a combination of materials that are either glued or melted together (Figure 6.2). This type of orthotic is used to improve weight transfer, to support and stabilize deformities of the foot and lower extremity, and to relieve pressure. Semirigid materials are the most frequently used in orthotics. Since these orthoses are more flexible than rigid orthotics, they require less precision in their manufacture. As described in other sections of this book, semirigid orthotics can be molded either directly to the foot or to a positive mold. The most popular materials used to fabricate semirigid orthotics are the cross-linked polyethylene foams, such as Plastazote, Aliplast, and Pelite, in firmer grades (Schwartz, 1991).

- Grade 1 density is 3 to 4 pounds per cubic foot, compression set 30 percent of thickness.

- Grade 2 density is 4.5 to 6 pounds per cubic foot, compression set 20 percent.

- Grade 3 density is 7 to 10 pounds per cubic foot, compression set 10 percent.

- Grade 4 density is 12 pounds per cubic foot, compression set less than 5 percent.

Nickelplast, another popular cross-linked polyethylene foam, has the advantage of high strength since it is alloyed with ethylene vinyl acetate. This toughness resists bottoming out as quickly as other polyethylene foams. Nickelplast has a rubber-like texture not found in the other polyethylene foams.

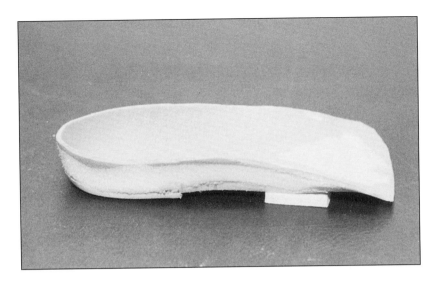

Figure 6.2 Semirigid orthotic of Aliplast and Plastazote.

When heated, Nickelplast shrinks about 15 percent, and upon cooling it becomes slightly harder. It comes in durometers (a measure of hardness) of 42 for Nickelplast-Lite, 45 for Nickelplast-S, and 55 for Nickelplast X-Firm. Nickelplast is moldable at 300 to 350 °F (150 to 175 °C) but does not readily autoadhere. Nickelplast should be glued when used with another material.

Ethylene vinyl acetate (EVA) is a polyolefin co-polymer that is often used as the midsole material of running shoes. It is thermoplastic but does not autoadhere. Heating for 3 to 5 minutes at 320 °F (160 °C) softens the material so that it may be formed. A small amount of shrinkage occurs with heating. EVA has two main uses in orthotics. Many practitioners use it for posting material either for the forefoot or the rearfoot. The other major use is as the "all-in-one orthotic" (Philips, 1990).

Cork has been much used in the past for orthotics but has lost some of its popularity with the advent of polyethylene foams. It may be used in its natural state or combined with other substances. Natural cork is lightweight and maintains its density, so that it retains 90 percent of its original thickness. To reduce cracking due to cork's limited flexibility, a rubber binder is often added. Natural cork and rubberized cork are most often used as the base material or arch filler for an orthotic. Jahss (1991) states that a cork filler for the arch of a polyethylene foam extends the life of the orthotic from 2 months to 6 months. A thermoplastic binder is often added to cork to make the cork heat moldable and autoadhering when heated to 275 °F (135 °C) for 2 to 3 minutes (Schwartz, 1991).

Rigid Materials

Rigid orthotics are used mainly to control subtalar pronation (Schwartz, 1991). These orthotics are not well suited for high-speed sports but may be used for walking and edge-control sports, such as skiing or skating (Subotnick, 1983). Most rigid orthoses are made from acrylic plastic or an acrylic plastic and carbon fiber composite (Sims & Cavanagh, 1991). The four most commonly used rigid orthotic plastics are polypropylene, laminated plastics, acrylics, and polyprolene (Jahss, 1991). These materials offer strength, durability, and hardness but have very limited flexibility. They are often made of only one layer of material (Schwartz, 1991). Functional rigid orthotics are made from a positive cast (Subotnick, 1975). Schwartz lists several drawbacks to the use of hard orthotics:

- Limited impact reduction

- Increased pressure areas

- High skill required to make them

- Materials often crack with high forces

- Special high-tech equipment required for fabrication (convection ovens, grinders, sanders, special saws, vacuum forming equipment, etc.)

- Contraindicated for persons with anesthetic areas, rigid deformities, or participation in high-impact sports

Kaye and Shereff (1991) list potential problems from rigid orthotics for high-mileage runners:

- Neuromas
- Nerve impingement
- Stress fractures
- Decreased shock absorption

Acrylic rigid orthotics are made mostly from polymers of polymethyl methacralate, a material originally used to cement hip and knee replacements firmly into place. Plexidure is a hard and rigid thermoplastic acrylic (Ferguson, Raskowsky, Blake, & Denton, 1991) (Figure 6.3). Its hardness and rigidity allow it to be used as an orthotic at thicknesses of 3.5 millimeters (slightly over 1/8 inch). This thinness is an obvious advantage for fit in a shallow shoe. Plexidure is heat moldable at approximately 350 °F (175 °C).

TL-61 is a composite plastic (a combination of different plastics into one material) that has gained recent popularity as an orthotic material (Schwartz, 1991). It was introduced in 1986 as a possible successor to Rohadur. It has the stiffness and durability of Rohadur but at only half the thickness. To achieve these qualities, TL-61 is composed of a heterogenous thermoplastic reinforced by a network of graphite fibers woven into the material. TL-61 is heat moldable, but grinding is not feasible on the surface or at an angle greater than 45 degrees on the edges due to weakening (Ferguson et al., 1991).

Aquaplast is a low-temperature thermoplastic polyester, rigid enough to be considered a hard orthotic material despite being heat moldable at 140 °F (60 °C). It has become a very popular choice of material among clinicians in recent years. It is autoadhering and may be re-formed with heat. Often, cold water is applied to speed cooling and setting. Available in various thicknesses, Aquaplast comes either perforated or nonperforated and is acrylic coated so that the surface will not bond instantly. Aquaplast will stretch with heat and traction. Different grades are color-coded to show the amount of elasticity. Green stripe has minimal stretch, while blue has maximal (Peppard & O'Donnell, 1983). A unique feature of Aquaplast is that it is transparent while warm and moldable, allowing easy observation of landmarks during the molding process.

Choice of Material

With such a wide range from which to choose, how does one select the proper material? The choice of material for fabrication is one of the first decisions to be made when orthotics are selected as a treatment regimen. Campbell et al. (1982) list nine properties to consider when choosing an orthotic material:

- Biocompatibility
- Ease of use
- Ease of fabrication
- Availability
- Durability
- Simulation of the mechanical properties of soft tissue
- Subjective comfort
- Cost
- Pressure-distributing properties

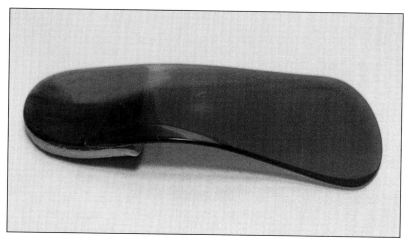

Figure 6.3 Rigid Plexidure orthotic.

In our practice the choice of orthotic materials is based on several factors:

- *Amount of control needed.* Obviously, a severe pronator will not receive the needed support with a soft orthotic. Some type of rigid or hard semirigid device will work best.

- *Activities of the individual.* From our review of the literature, it is worth noting that many authors feel that rigid orthotics are not the first choice for the high-level athlete participating in sprinting and cutting sports.

- *Foot type.* The literature suggests that foot type is an important indicator of the type of orthotic best suited for an individual. The high-arched foot is rigid and needs a more flexible and cushioned device. Flat feet are not as easily categorized as to the type of orthotic needed.

- *Medical indications.* Certainly people with diabetes, people with rheumatoid arthritis, and other individuals with special needs require specialized materials with properties suited to their problems.

- *Type of shoe an individual plans to use the orthotics in.* Shoes with increased depth and width will allow larger devices, whereas heels and many women's shoes require an ultra-thin device.

Covers

Most orthotics are covered with a lining as the final step of the fabrication process. These linings provide a slightly rougher surface than the plastic to prevent slippage and add a small amount of cushion to the device. Linings also reduce the drop-off at the end of the orthotic, providing a transition between the end of the orthotic and the start of the shoe.

One of the most commonly used cover materials is Spenco, a rubber mix infused with nitrogen gas under pressure (Schwartz, 1991). Spenco has many uses and comes in various thicknesses. When used as an orthotic, Spenco has a top layer of stretch fabric.

Alicover is another popular covering material, consisting of Aliplast 4E at 1/16-inch thickness bonded to a six-way stretch nylon. Alicover may be glued or bonded to other pieces of Aliplast or Plastazote (Figure 6.4).

Full-length covers are invaluable for rectifying small problems with the orthotic fit. High edges, drop-off on the distal edge, and slippage all respond favorably to the simple addition of a full length cover. If a full-length cover is not readily available (for example, the patient is from out of town and experiences problems), then a flat insole may be used. Insoles can be purchased in most running stores. It is important to warn the patient that the insole should not have a built-in arch; it should be flat. The insole is either glued or taped onto the top of the orthotic. A temporary way to attach the insole to the orthotic is to loop the tape, sticky side out, and place it on the top of the device at the heel and at the forefoot.

Equipment

Appropriate equipment types and costs depend on the type and quantity of orthotics being made. Equipment may be simple and cheap if the number of orthotics being fabricated is not too large. As orthotic types become more complicated and numbers increase, then the need for more sophisticated equipment becomes important.

Ovens

Although any source of heat will theoretically be sufficient for orthotic fabrication, a convection

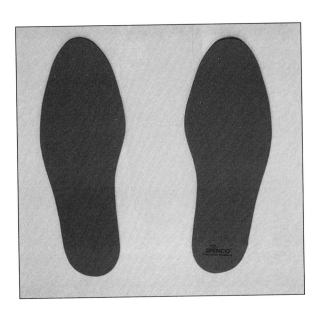

Figure 6.4 Orthotic cover of Aliplast.

oven is the best method of heating. Convection ovens provide an even distribution of heat to the material, which prevents the material from becoming too hot in one spot and not hot enough in another. Convection ovens may be purchased through almost any electric appliance store. As for size, the commonly used oven shown in Figure 6.5 measures 17 inches (425 mm) wide on the inside.

Grinders

A drum grinder is necessary to bevel edges and finish the bottom of the orthotic. The grinding surface must be wide enough, at least as wide as the bottom of the orthotic when it is pressed against the wheel. Three inches (75 mm) is about the minimum width. The Sani-Grinder, one of the more popular models, has a 3-inch wheel diameter with a 3-inch face. It has a two-speed motor (1,725 or 3,450 rpm) and comes with its own vacuum and bag, which is important due to the amount of debris created during grinding (see Figure 6.5). Red Wing is another popular brand of grinder. These and similar grinders may be found at dental or orthotic supply houses.

Formers

Vacuum formers may be used to mold the orthotic to the positive mold. There are various sizes and types (Figure 6.6). For those who do not make enough orthotics for a vacuum former to be feasible, a manual former may be an alternative.

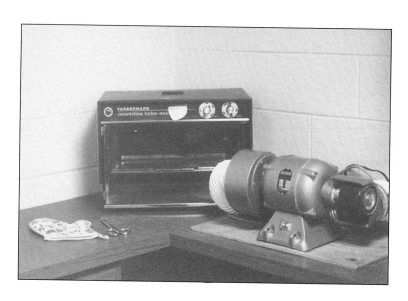

Figure 6.5 Convection oven, drum grinder with vacuum, large scissors, and heat-resistant mitt.

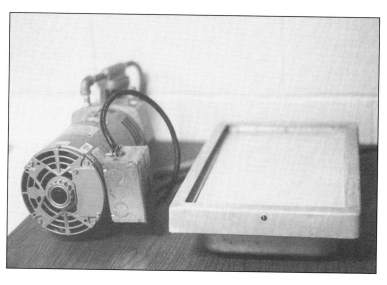

Figure 6.6 Vacuum former.

Placing an orthotic on the limb or mold without the use of a vacuum is called draping (Peppard & O'Donnell, 1983). A manual press may be used to mold the heated orthotic material firmly to the positive. The orthotic may also be held firmly against the positive by a binding piece of cloth (Ace wrap) or leather (Figure 6.7).

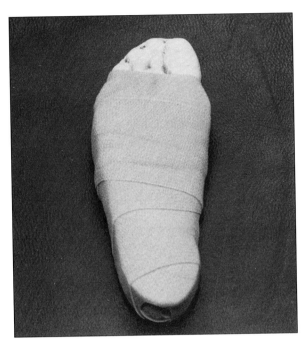

Figure 6.7   Ace wrap holding orthotic to positive.

Scissors

A large pair of scissors is necessary for the fabrication of an orthotic. Small bandage-type scissors are not able to cut all types of thermoplastic materials. Industrial scissors with a blade of at least 8 inches (20 cm) work the best.

Other Items

Other items are helpful when making any type of orthotic. Gloves that are heat resistant but allow some tactile sensation will be useful in handling hot orthotic material as it comes out of the oven. Safety glasses that fully protect the eyes are crucial while grinding. A surgical mask is also suggested during grinding to prevent inhalation of any orthotic material dust that escapes the vacuum.

Costs

The initial startup cost of this equipment and material has been estimated at $1,200 (McPoil & Brocato, 1985). AliMed, Inc. offers a complete startup kit, including oven, grinder, scissors, heat gun, and several types of thermoplastics, for $1,071 (1994 catalog).

Summary

A variety of materials and equipment may be used in the manufacture of orthotics. The practitioner may use patient factors such as activity, foot type, diagnosis and severity of problem, and shoe dimensions to guide the decision about which materials and equipment to use. The physical properties of various orthotic materials may also be a factor in this decision.

References

Campbell, G., Newell, E., & McLure, M. (1982). Compression testing of foamed plastics and rubbers for use as orthotic shoe insoles. *Prosthetics and Orthotics International*, **6**, 48–52.

Cracchiolo, A. (1982). Office treatment of adult foot problems. *Orthopedic Clinics of North America*, **13**, 511.

Enna, C., Brand, P., Reed, J., & Welch, D. (1976). The orthotic care of the denervated foot in Hansen's disease. *Orthotics and Prosthetics*, **30**, 33–39.

Ferguson, H., Raskowsky, M., Blake, R., & Denton, J. (1991). TL-61 versus Rohadur orthoses in heel spur syndrome. *Journal of the American Podiatric Medical Association*, **81**, 439–442.

Gere, J., & Timoshenko, S. (1984). *Mechanics of material*. Boston: PWS/Kent.

Glass, M., Karno, M., Sella, E., & Zeleznik, R. (1982). An office based orthotic system in treatment of the arthritic foot. *Foot and Ankle*, **3**, 37–40.

Gould, J. (1982). Conservative management of the hypersensitive foot in rheumatoid arthritis. *Foot and Ankle*, **2**, 224–227.

Hertzman, C. (1973). Use of Plastazote in foot disabilities. *American Journal of Physical Medicine*, **52**, 289–303.

Holmes, D. (1980). Orthotics of the foot and ankle. In A. Helfet & D. Grubel-Lee (Eds.), *Disorders of the foot* (pp. 228–233). Philadelphia: Lippincott.

Jahss, M. (1991). Arch supports, shielding, and orthodigita. In M. Jahss (Ed.), *Disorders of the foot and ankle* (pp. 2857–2865). Philadelphia: Saunders.

Kaye, R., & Shereff, M. (1991). Athletic footwear, modifications, and orthotic devices. In M. Jahss (Ed.), *Disorders of the foot and ankle* (pp. 2910–2920). Philadelphia: Saunders.

McPoil, T.G., & Brocato, R.S. (1985). The foot and ankle: Biomechanical evaluation and treatment. In S. Gould & G. Davies (Eds.), *Orthopedic and Sports Physical Therapy* (p. 314). St. Louis: Mosby.

Murphy, E., & Burnstein, A. (1975). Physical properties of materials including solid mechanics. In American Academy of Orthopedic Surgeons (Eds.), *Atlas of orthotics* (pp. 3–30). St. Louis: Mosby.

Olson, W. (1988). Orthoses: An analysis of their component materials. *Journal of the American Podiatric Medical Association*, **78**, 203.

Peppard, A., & O'Donnell, M. (1983). A review of orthotic plastics. *Athletic Training*, **18**, 77–80.

Philips, J. (1990). *The functional foot orthosis.* New York: Churchill Livingstone.

Rome, K. (1990). Behavior of orthotic materials in chiropody. *Journal of the American Podiatric Medical Association*, **80**, 471–477.

Rome, K. (1991). A study of the properties of materials used in podiatry. *Journal of the American Podiatric Medical Association*, **81**, 73–83.

Schwartz, R. (1991). Foot orthoses and materials. In M. Jahss (Ed.), *Disorders of the foot and ankle* (pp. 2866–2878). Philadelphia: Saunders.

Showers, D., & Strunck, M. (1985). Sheet plastics and their applications in orthotics and prosthetics. *Orthotics and Prosthetics*, **38**, 41–48.

Sims, D., & Cavanagh, P. (1991). Selected foot mechanics related to the prescription of foot orthoses. In M. Jahss (Ed.), *Disorders of the foot and ankle* (pp. 469–483). Philadelphia: Saunders.

Subotnick, S. (1975). *Podiatric sports medicine.* Mt. Kisco, NY: Futura.

Subotnick, S. (1983). Foot orthoses: An update. *The Physician and Sportsmedicine*, **11**, 103–106.

White, F. (1992). Orthotics. In J. Drennan (Ed.), *The child's foot and ankle* (p. 72). New York: Raven Press.

In-Office Fabrication of Semirigid Orthotics

7

The advantages of in-office fabrication of temporary semirigid orthotics are many, but the greatest is the decreased time demand on the patient. It is possible, using the technique described by Donovan et al. (1979) and Kuland, Soos, and Vannoy (1979), to fabricate devices in 60 to 90 minutes as opposed to the several days or weeks waiting for return mail from a laboratory. The in-office devices are comfortable, inexpensive (less than $10 per pair for materials), adjustable, and effective. Their durability is limited, depending on the size and activity level of the patient. Service life for foot orthotics may range from 6 to 18 months.

For patients needing a high level of motion control, rigid plastic is the material of choice. For patients needing less motion control and a reduction in the forces acting at the foot and lower extremity, temporary semirigid thermoplastic devices have been shown to be effective.

The technique of fabrication, developed by Dr. Rob Roy McGreger in 1972, incorporates the use of foamed thermoplastics, specifically Plastazote and Aliplast (Donovan et al., 1979). These plastics are heated in a convection oven, molded to the patient's foot, trimmed, ground, and posted according to the patient's needs. The success of this operation is dependent on a careful evaluation of the lower quarter and the skill of the person fabricating the orthotics. Cutting and grinding the material require highly coordinated fine motor skills and confidence in the use of power tools. Proficiency can only be gained through practice.

General Fabrication Technique

In this description of orthotic fabrication, Aliplast 0, Buff (1/8-in. thickness), and Plastazote 2 (1/4-in. thickness) are used. These materials are available from AliMed, Inc.

With all the needed materials gathered and the oven preheated to 285 °F (140 °C), the patient's foot is placed on a sheet of 1/8-inch Aliplast. Draw a rectangle around the foot, leaving a margin of at least 1/2 inch (13 mm) from the heel and great toe (Figure 7.1). Cut along the outline, and cut a matching piece of Plastazote (Figure 7.2). These pieces are placed in the oven, with the Plastazote against the supporting grate (Figure 7.3). If the Aliplast is placed against hot metal, it will adhere and burn. The thermoplastics, which take approximately 4 minutes to soften, should be checked regularly to prevent overheating and to flatten any air pockets.

If a deep heel cup is desired in the orthotic (in treating plantar fasciitis), it is preferable to mold the thermoplastic with the patient prone, the knee flexed 90 degrees, the ankle in neutral, and the foot protected with a thin sock or stockinette (Figure 7.4). Before the plastic can be molded to the patient's foot, the subtalar neutral position must be determined. Neutral position is approximated by palpating the head of the talus (Figure 7.5). With neutral determined, molding can begin when the thermoplastic is soft, pliable, and free of air bubbles. The thermoplastic is removed from the oven with gloved hands and is placed over the

Cutting and Heating the Materials

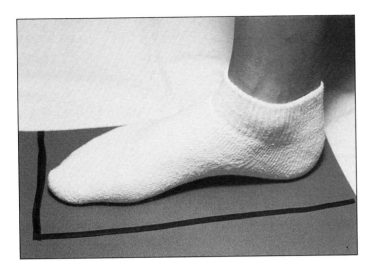

Figure 7.1 Place foot on Aliplast, and cut a rectangle with 1/2-inch (13 millimeter) borders.

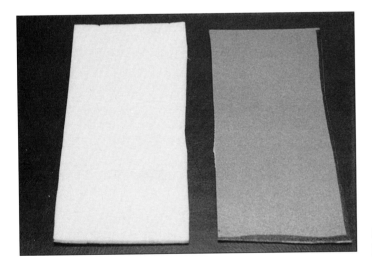

Figure 7.2 Cut a matching piece of Plastazote.

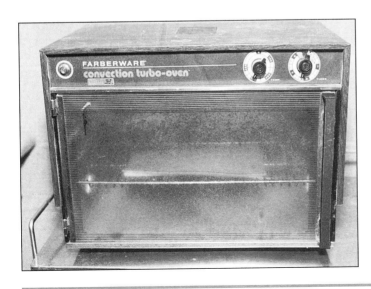

Figure 7.3 Place the Aliplast in the oven with the Plastazote against the supporting grate.

Molding the Plastic to the Foot

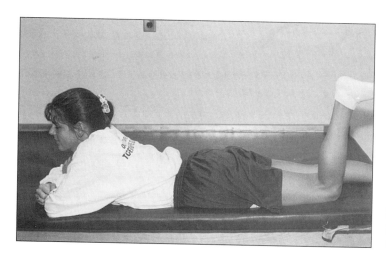

Figure 7.4 Patient is positioned in prone position; the knee is flexed to 90 degrees to facilitate a deep heel cup.

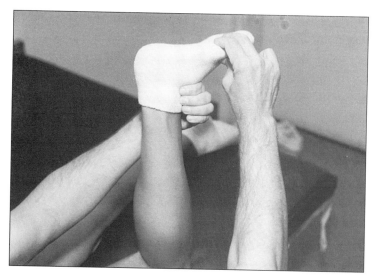

Figure 7.5 Determining neutral subtalar joint position.

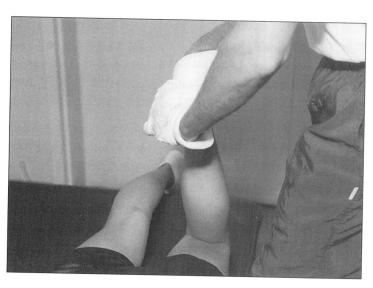

Figure 7.6 Thermoplastic material is removed from the oven and molded over the patient's foot.

foot. The operator places one hand over the heel and one over the arch and applies gentle pressure to capture the contour of the foot (Figure 7.6). The plastic is held in this position for 1 minute. The procedure is repeated on the opposite foot.

Next, with the patient sitting, an outline of the foot is traced in the plastic (Figure 7.7). The outline crosses the front of the foot at the level of the toe sulcus (Figure 7.8).

An alternative method of molding the plastic can be completed with the patient seated. This method produces a flat-bottomed orthotic that is easier to post and grind. The patient is seated with knee flexed 90 degrees, ankle in neutral, and sock-

protected foot on the casting pillow (Figure 7.9). Neutral is determined by palpating the talar head (Figure 7.10). The plastic is removed from the oven with gloved hands and placed on the casting pillow. The foot is placed on the plastic with one hand maintaining neutral and the other hand reinforcing the arch (Figure 7.11, a and b). The patient is instructed to press down slightly. The greater the pressure, the deeper the heel cup and arch, and the harder to maintain subtalar neutral. After 1 minute, the foot is traced on the plastic, and the outline trimmed (Figure 7.12). The patient can now relax and wait while the devices are ground and posted.

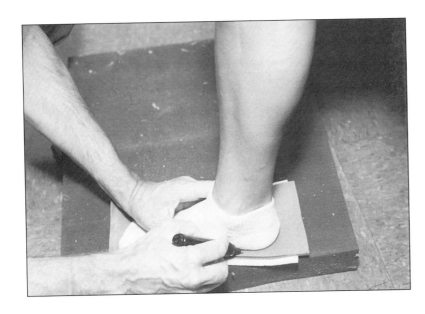

Figure 7.7 Patient is seated, and an outline of the foot is traced onto the material.

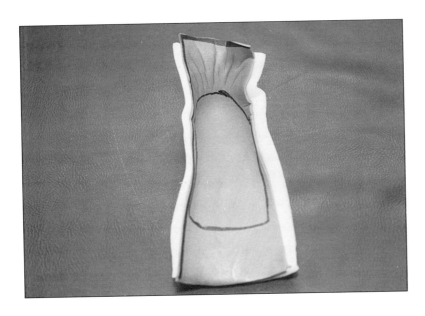

Figure 7.8 The outline crosses the front of the foot at the level of the toe sulcus.

Molding the Plastic With the Patient Seated

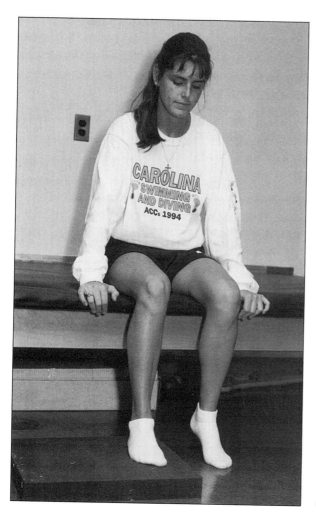

Figure 7.9 Seated position for orthotic fabrication.

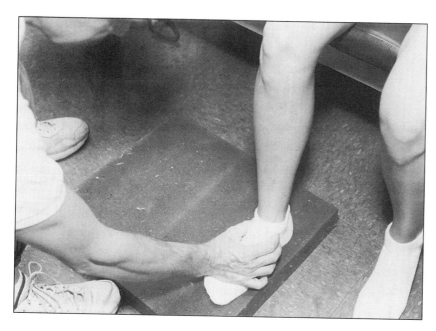

Figure 7.10 Determining subtalar neutral position in seated position.

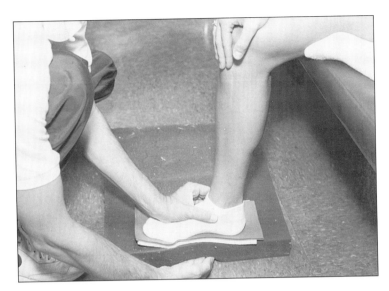

Figure 7.11 Material is molded to the patient's foot. Note position of the hand molding the arch.

a

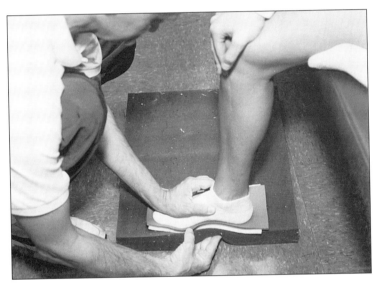

b

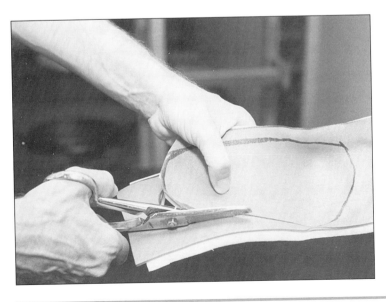

Figure 7.12 Trim along the marked outline.

Grinding produces plastic dust necessitating the use of eye protection, a mask to cover the nose and mouth, and appropriate covering of the operator's clothing. Care must be taken to avoid hand and finger contact with the grinding wheel since severe lacerations and abrasions can occur. The more familiar the operator is with the grinder, the more proficient the finished fabrication. The initial grind is a bevel of approximately 20 degrees around the outside edge of the orthotic (Figure 7.13). This bevel may be cut deeper under the arch and at the heel. This grinding allows the device to fit snugly in the shoe. Next, the front of the orthotic is ground back to the level of the metatarsal heads, marked prior to grinding (Figure 7.14, a & b).

The bottom of the orthotic is ground flat, with the bottom of the heel being ground first and then the forefoot relative to the heel (Figure 7.15). An experienced operator can incorporate some posting with these grinds. Care must be taken not to grind through the device at the heel or to leave the area too thin. Figure 7.16 compares a finished device on the right and an unfinished on the left. Note the beveled edges, the forefoot ground to the level of the metatarsal heads, and the flattened heel with Aliplast exposed. Figure 7.17 compares the finished and unfinished orthotics as seen from behind. Note the flattened heel and beveled edges.

Grinding the Orthotic

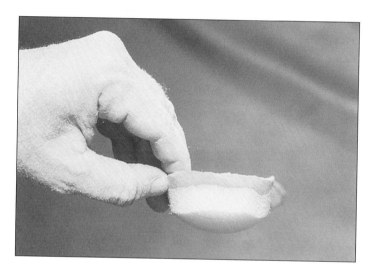

Figure 7.13 Initial grind is approximately 20 degrees around the outside of the orthotic.

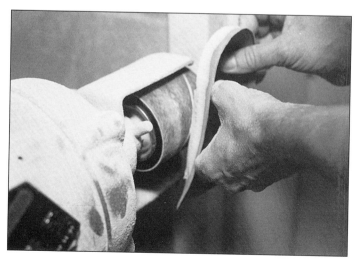

Figure 7.14 The orthotic is ground back (a) to the premarked level of the metatarsal heads (b).

a

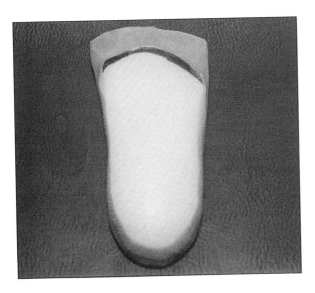

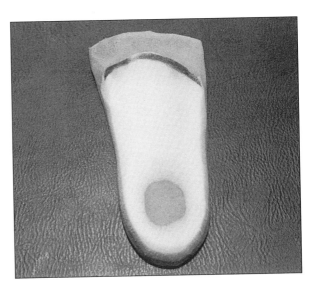

Figure 7.14b

Figure 7.15   The bottom of the orthotic is ground flat.

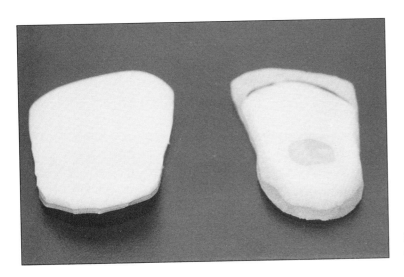

Figure 7.16   Finished and unfinished orthotics.

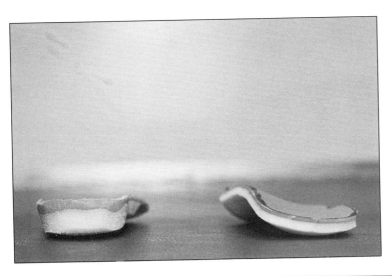

Figure 7.17   Finished and unfinished orthotic seen from rear.

Fabricating the device to the toe sulcus rather than the metatarsal heads prevents the orthotic from migrating in the shoe. Firm positioning in the shoe is especially important for athletes in sports that require lateral movement, such as tennis and basketball. In many cases, additional support under the arch and posting will be needed. To support the arch, cut a piece of 1/4-inch Plastazote to fit the arch of the orthotic (Figure 7.18) and heat in the oven long enough to soften it slightly. Mold to the arch. Mark the support's outline on the orthotic, and coat the adjoining surfaces with contact cement (Figure 7.19). The pieces are pressed together tightly (Figure 7.20). The additional arch material is then ground, first to match the bevels on the edge and then to flatten the bottom (Figure 7.21). Figure 7.22 shows the device with the arch support attached.

Creating the Arch Support

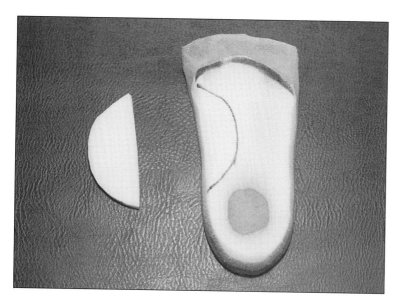

Figure 7.18 Plastazote added to support the arch.

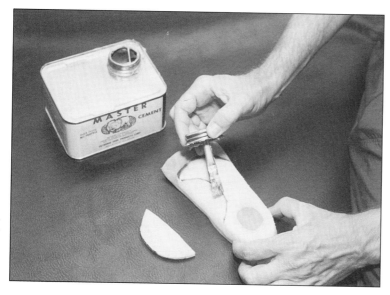

Figure 7.19 Contact cement is applied to the orthotic and arch support.

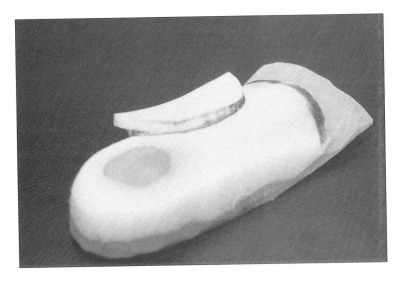

Figure 7.20   Applying the arch support to the orthotic.

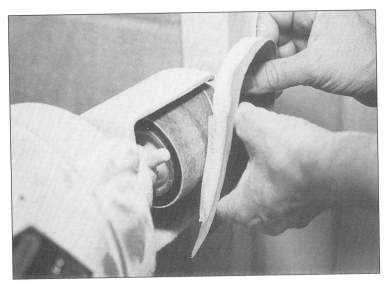

Figure 7.21   Grinding the arch-support material to flatten the bottom.

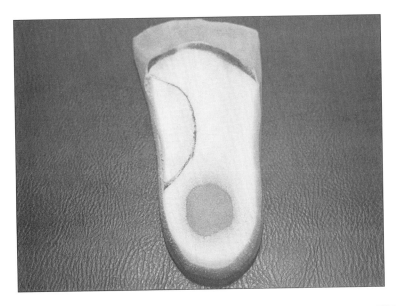

Figure 7.22   Orthotic with arch support attached.

Modifications for Specific Concerns

If the area under the heel is ground too thin, an additional piece of 1/8-inch Aliplast can be used to support this area (Figure 7.23, a & b). Heat a piece of Aliplast approximately the size of the heel, and mold over the heel of the device. When heated, Aliplast must be placed in a piece of pasteboard to prevent the plastic from adhering to the oven. After molding, the Aliplast is glued to the heel. Similarly, heel lifts can be fabricated by adding layers of Aliplast to achieve the desired height.

A horseshoe-shaped heel pad provides pain relief from heel spurs, stone bruises, and plantar fasciitis. In fabrication of a horseshoe-shaped pad, a small piece of thermoplastic material is heated, molded, traced, cut, and then glued to the heel (Figure 7.24). Aliplast, Nickelplast, and Poron all work well for this procedure.

Posting is accomplished using either 1/8-inch Aliplast or Nickelplast. This thickness allows approximately 4 to 6 degrees of posting; higher degrees can be achieved by adding more material. Pictured in Figure 7.25 are Nickelplast pieces cut and traced for medial forefoot and rearfoot posts. These are glued to the orthotic and then ground to the desired angle (Figure 7.26).

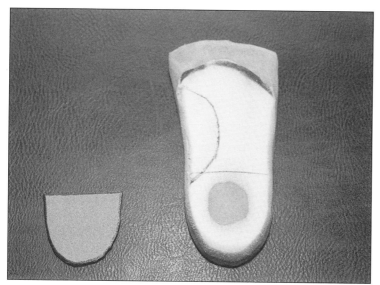

Figure 7.23   If the orthotic heel is ground too thin, an additional piece of Aliplast (a) may be added (b).

a

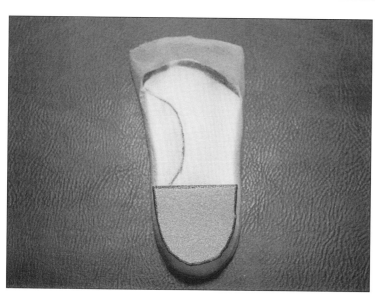

b

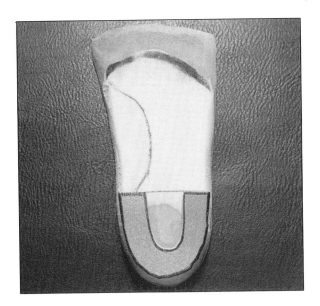

Figure 7.24 A horseshoe pad added to the bottom of an orthotic.

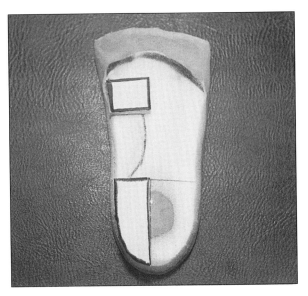

Figure 7.25 Nickelplast cut for forefoot and rearfoot posts.

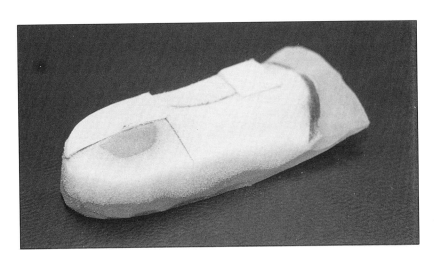

Figure 7.26 Forefoot and rearfoot posts after grinding.

A Nickelplast teardrop pad provides support for the metatarsal arch. The pad is cut (Figure 7.27) and the edges beveled prior to affixing the pad to the orthotic temporarily with tape. The patient walks for 2 or 3 minutes to determine if the pad placement is correct. When the correct position is found, the pad is glued in place (Figure 7.28). A metatarsal bar is fabricated in a similar manner using 1/8-inch Aliplast but is ground after being glued to the device (Figures 7.29 & 7.30).

Relief for a patient with sesamoiditis is provided by either a crescent-shaped pad placed just behind the sesamoids or by cutting and grinding of the orthotic device under the first metatarsal head. The purpose of both techniques is to prevent weightbearing under the sesamoids. A crescent-shaped pad is cut from 1/8-inch Nickelplast and glued just proximal to the first metatarsal joint (Figure 7.31). If this technique is not successful, then trim and grind the orthotic under the first metatarsal to move weightbearing in a proximal direction from the sesamoids (Figure 7.32).

Patients with extremely high arches require more support than can be accomplished by building up the bottom of the orthotic. Additional support for the arch can be provided with 1/4-inch Plastazote glued to the top of the orthotic. The Plastazote is cut to two-thirds of the width of the foot and the length of the longitudinal arch and heated until pliable. The material is placed on the casting pillow (Figure 7.33) and the sock-protected foot is placed on top. The foot is maintained in

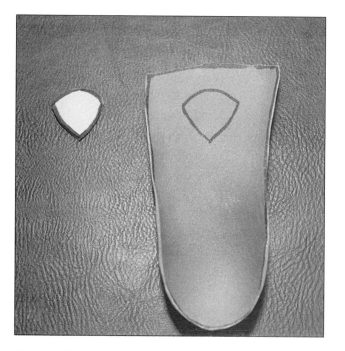

Figure 7.27 A Nickelplast teardrop pad.

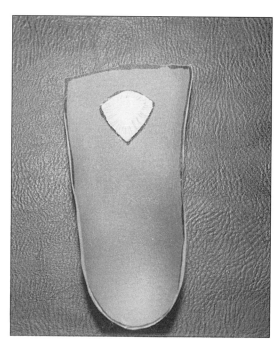

Figure 7.28 The teardrop pad glued in place.

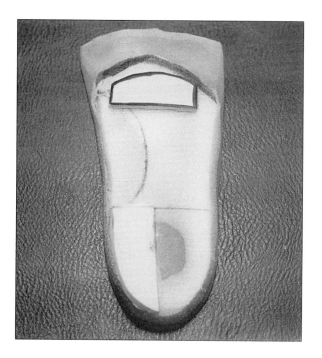

Figure 7.29 A metatarsal bar cut and added to the bottom of an orthotic.

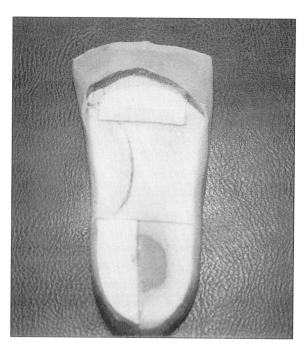

Figure 7.30 The metatarsal bar is ground after being added to the device.

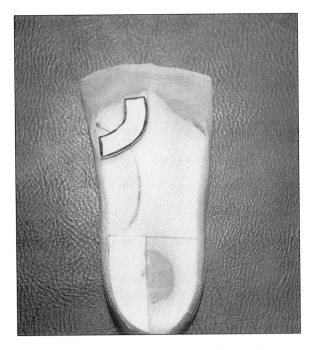

Figure 7.31 A crescent-shaped pad added to the orthotic to relieve sesamoiditis.

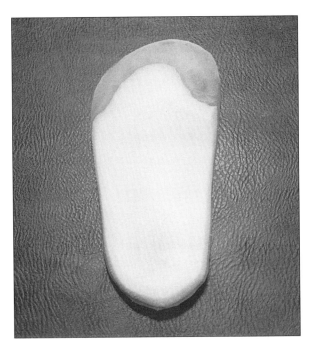

Figure 7.32 The orthotic ground under the first metatarsal to decrease weightbearing on the sesamoids.

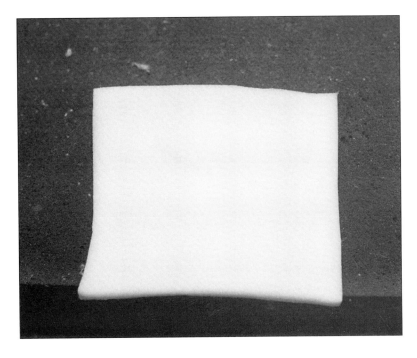

Figure 7.33 A heated piece of Plastazote on the casting block, preparatory to adding material to the top of the orthotic.

subtalar neutral and the arch is supported as the thermoplastic is molded (Figure 7.34). This high-arch support is then trimmed and ground to bevel the edges. Proper alignment is determined by first taping the additional arch support in place and having the patient walk for 2 or 3 minutes (Figure 7.35). When proper alignment is determined, the support is traced in

place on the orthotic and glued. After gluing, the outside edge is ground to match the bevel and height of the orthotic (Figure 7.36).

A covering of Spenco or PPT can be added as a finishing touch (Figure 7.37, a & b). The cover adds cushioning and helps provide a tight fit if the original insole has been removed from the shoe.

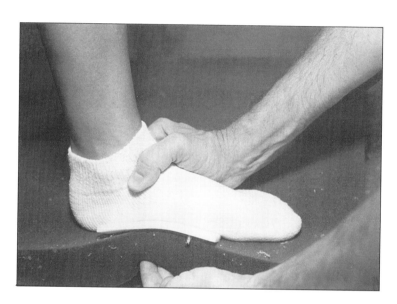

Figure 7.34 While maintained in neutral, the foot is placed on the material, which is then molded.

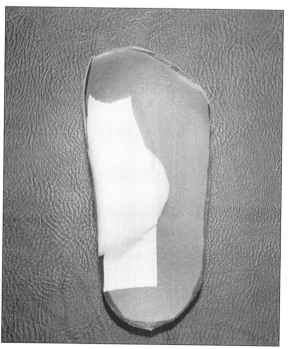

Figure 7.35 Tape the high-arch support onto the orthotic. Before gluing, allow the patient to walk to find the optimal position for the support.

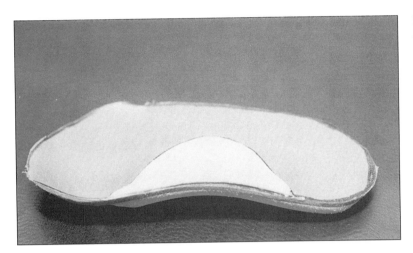

Figure 7.36 Glue the support to the top of the device, and grind the outside edge of the support to match the bevel and height of the orthotic.

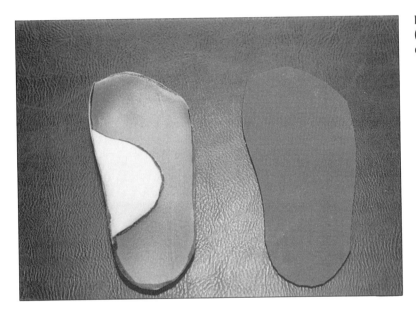

Figure 7.37 Covering material (a) added to the top of the orthotic device (b).

a

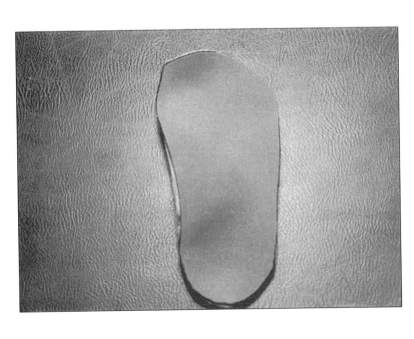

b

Summary

The effectiveness of orthotics produced in the office is dependent upon the skill of the clinician in evaluating the biomechanics of the lower quarter and then translating this information into an effective device. Practice and patience are needed to develop the skill to position the patient properly, mold the thermoplastics, and then grind and adjust the finished devices. If successful, the result is an effective, comfortable, convenient, and inexpensive pair of orthotics.

References

Donovan, J.C., Scardina, R.J., & Frykberg, R.G., Hill, C.E., & Lucchini, E. (1979). New England Deaconess Hospital Podiatry Service—sport orthotic device. *Journal of the American Podiatry Association*, **69**(9), 571–574.

Kuland, D., Soos, T., & Vannoy, P. (1979). Airplane insulation for flying feet. *Athletic Training*, **14**(3).

Rigid Orthotics

8

This chapter will discuss fabrication techniques for rigid orthotics. As stated previously, we seldom fabricate rigid orthotics in our clinical setting because of the complexity and time-consuming nature of the process. For completeness, this chapter on rigid foot orthotics is included.

The decision to fabricate the rigid orthotic in-house must be based on the availability of the proper equipment and the expertise of the clinician. The clinician must be aware of the amount of heat needed to make the thermoplastics workable and how much heat is absorbed by the material. This information is critical to ensure that the material can be applied to the positive mold successfully. As information resources, Combs-Orteza, Vogelbach, and Denegar (1992), Doxey (1985), and Lutter (1980) have described fabrication methods for rigid to semirigid devices. We also recommend the textbooks by Anthony (1991) and Philips (1990).

Having a Laboratory Manufacture the Orthotic

When a rigid orthotic is indicated, we typically use a set of temporary orthotics to determine if they are an appropriate aspect of the total rehabilitation process of the patient. The use of the temporary orthotics also allows the clinician to fine-tune and make adjustments to the device, incorporating feedback from the patient (Donatelli, Hurlbert, Conaway, & St. Pierre, 1988).

Initially, a negative cast of the foot in neutral subtalar joint position is taken, as described in chapter 5. The cast is then packaged and shipped to an orthotic laboratory with the information from the biomechanical examination so that the proper posting measurements and specifications are incorporated into the orthotic device. An alternative to the cast method is the use of foam impression trays to capture the foot in neutral subtalar joint position, also described in chapter 5. The tray is then packaged and shipped to the laboratory.

Manufacturing an Orthotic From a Positive Mold In-House

Manufacturing a rigid or semirigid orthotic in-house from a positive mold will require additional time and equipment. However, many clinicians find this process very challenging and rewarding. Indeed, skilled practitioners can fabricate an excellent device at a fraction of the cost of having orthotics made in a laboratory. In addition, having the proper equipment and materials allows a rigid orthotic to be modified in-house if it is not providing its intended function.

Modification of the Positive Mold

Philips (1990) and Anthony (1991) describe in detail the methods of modifying the positive mold to correct structural or positional deformities of the foot. This process includes shaping, augmenting with added material, sanding, and grinding of the mold before the orthotic is fabricated. Darrigan and Ganley (1985) describe a method in which screws are inserted into the positive mold and additional plaster applied to correct forefoot deformity. Colonna (1989) describes a similar technique used in the fabrication of semirigid devices. Modification of a positive mold is a time-consuming and demanding task that can only be successfully completed with the proper expertise and equipment.

Fabrication From a Positive Mold

After the positive mold has been modified to compensate for structural or positional imbalances of the foot and lower kinetic chain, the orthotic can be fabricated. After the appropriate material has been chosen, a piece slightly larger than the anticipated orthosis is heated and molded over the positive mold. Rigid material is pressed onto the modified positive mold using a hand or vacuum press, as illustrated in Figure 8.1. Some rigid materials can be satisfactorily molded to the positive by hand, but we recommend some type of pressing procedure or vacuum apparatus for better results (Brown & Smith, 1976). The posting of this type of orthotic is intrinsic, as the corrections have already been made to the positive mold, especially at the forefoot (Darrigan & Ganley, 1985). Again, this type of orthotic fabrication requires expertise in mold modification and significant amounts of time. The use of this type of rigid material and method of fabrication allows for little to no modification of the orthotic once it has been made, thereby necessitating exact measurements and orthotic prescription.

Prefabricated Shells

Another option in rigid orthotics is to purchase prefabricated shells from a distributor. The shells come in sizes that correspond to shoe sizes (Figure 8.2). The shell can be heated and then molded over the positive mold. If the positive has been modified, then intrinsic posting is incorporated in the orthotic as it hardens. The clinician may choose to press prefabricated shells onto a positive mold that has not been modified, as illustrated in Figure 8.3. In this case, extrinsic posts are added to the orthotics to correct for structural deformities. Extrinsic posting requires use of material that is suitably rigid, such as dental acrylics, and that will bond to the rigid thermoplastic (see Figure 8.4). Prefabricated shells can be modified by heating, as with a heat gun, to change the arch or metatarsal lift incorporated into the orthotic device. The clinician must wear insulated gloves to prevent burns.

Fabrication Directly Onto the Patient's Foot

Rigid or semirigid orthotic shells can be molded directly onto the patient's foot. The foot is maintained in neutral subtalar joint position with the midtarsal joint in a pronated position, as described by Doxey (1985), and Combs-Orteza, Vogelbach, and Denegar (1992). The patient is placed in either the supine or prone position, depending on the preference of the clinician. Depending on the physical properties of the material being used, the patient's foot may need to be insulated and monitored for excessive heat buildup. Heated to the recommended temperature, the material

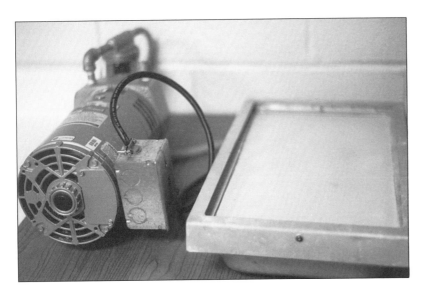

Figure 8.1 Use a vacuum press to mold the heated rigid material to the positive mold.

Using Prefabricated Shells

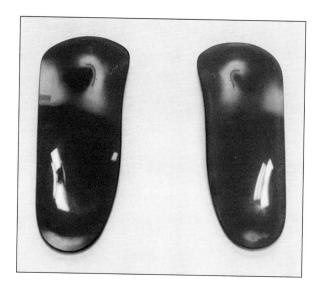

Figure 8.2 Prefabricated rigid orthotic shells.

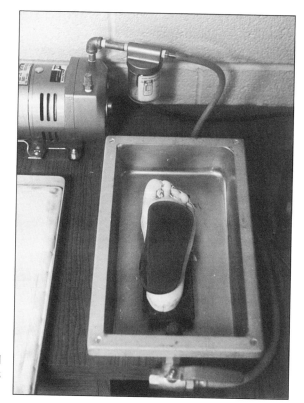

Figure 8.3 Pressing prefabricated shells onto a positive mold that has not been modified.

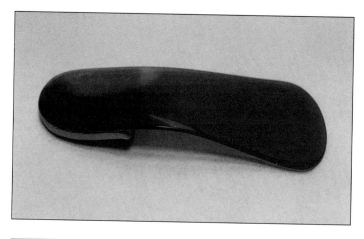

Figure 8.4 Extrinsic forefoot and rearfoot posts added to a rigid shell.

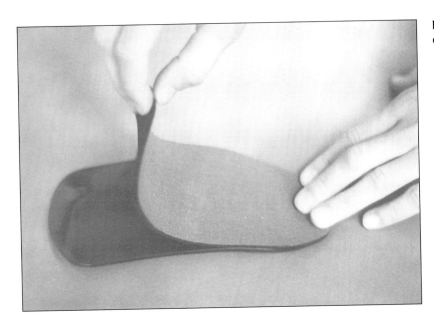

Figure 8.5 Application of a top cover to the rigid orthotic device.

should be molded from the calcaneus to the metatarsals. After the shell has cooled, the appropriate extrinsic forefoot and rearfoot posts are applied and modified by the use of a grinder or appropriate tools. These types of orthotics usually require a top cover to increase the friction between the foot and the usually slick surface of the thermoplastic to prevent sliding (Figure 8.5).

Summary

Rigid orthotics are indicated for patients who need absolute biomechanical control of abnormal subtalar and midtarsal joint movements. They require modification of the positive mold into which the rigid material is pressed. Therefore the posts are usually intrinsic. Modification is very difficult if the negative cast or positive molds have been incorrectly fabricated. Rigid orthotic fabrication is time-consuming and requires specialized skills. Most physical therapy and athletic training settings are not equipped or staffed to produce rigid orthotics. When indicated, we use an orthotic laboratory or refer patients to a podiatrist.

References

Anthony, R.J. (1991). *The manufacture and use of the functional foot orthosis.* Basel: Karger.

Brown, D., & Smith, C. (1976). Vacuum casting for foot orthoses. *Journal of the American Podiatry Association, 66*, 582–587.

Colonna, P. (1989). Fabrication of a custom molded orthotic using an intrinsic posting technique for a forefoot varus deformity. *Physical Therapy Forum, 8*, 6–7.

Combs-Orteza, L., Vogelbach, D.W., & Denegar, C.R. (1992). The effect of molded and unmolded orthotics on balance and pain while jogging following inversion ankle sprain. *Journal of Athletic Training, 27*, 80–84.

Darrigan, R.D., & Ganley, J.V. (1985). Functional orthoses with intrinsic rearfoot posting. *Journal of the American Podiatric Medical Association, 75*, 619–625.

Donatelli, R., Hurlbert, C., Conaway, D., & St. Pierre, R. (1988). Biomechanical foot orthotics: A retrospective study. *The Journal of Orthopaedic and Sports Physical Therapy, 10*, 205–212.

Doxey, G.E. (1985). Clinical use and fabrication of molded thermoplastic foot orthotic devices. *Physical Therapy, 65*, 1679–1682.

Lutter, L.D. (1980). Foot-related knee problems in the long distance runner. *Foot and Ankle, 1*, 112–116.

Philips, J.W. (1990). *The functional foot orthosis.* New York: Churchill Livingstone.

Orthotics for Special Conditions

9

Not every patient needs a standard orthotic. Certain orthopedic conditions are best treated with special adaptations to regular orthotics. These modifications may be in the form of extensions to the length of the orthotic, increased depth of the device, areas of relief or prominence built into the orthotic, or the use of different materials better adapted to needs of the individual.

Many adaptations originally designed for special populations may be useful in other applications as well. For example, soft orthotics are often prescribed for severe metatarsalgia but are also used frequently for rheumatoid arthritis.

Adaptations for special problems require a thorough knowledge of the etiology of the problem as well as a thorough working knowledge of orthotics. One must conquer the basics of orthotic fabrication before attempting any adaptation. It is important to remember that these special orthotics are not meant to be standard orthotics and should be reserved for special problems demanding more than the normal orthotic treatment plan. This chapter will discuss the treatment of various problems requiring a modification of the standard orthotic.

The Rheumatoid Foot

This discussion of orthotic devices for rheumatoid arthritis is intended for those clinicians whose educational backgrounds include management of these patients. Referral to podiatrists or orthotists may be necessary in complicated cases.

Foot problems may occur in up to 90 percent of rheumatoid patients (Coughlin, 1984). Problems in the rheumatoid foot usually manifest as synovial inflammation and proliferation. The proliferating synovium distends ligaments, resulting in instability and disfigurement of the joints of the foot. The affected synovium also limits nutrition of the articular cartilage of the joint, causing degeneration. As the synovium attacks the ligaments and tendons, adhesions occur. The most common site for any of these problems is the metatarsophalangeal joints of the foot. Orthotics are used to decrease plantar shear, provide more total contact, eliminate or shift contact in certain areas, and support unstable joints (Gould, 1982).

The principles used in constructing a soft orthotic for the rheumatoid foot are the same as for the diabetic or peripheral vascular foot (Glass, Karno, Sella, & Zeleznik, 1982). Many of the techniques used to treat the rheumatoid foot and the diabetic foot were first developed to treat leprosy (Hertzman, 1973; Mondl, Gardiner, & Bissett, 1969). A device similar to the rheumatoid foot orthotic is also recommended for many sports injuries (Hannaford, 1986). Plastazote is the most common material to treat these problems (Glass et al., 1982).

Our fabrication technique for rheumatoid and similar problems differs from the techniques already described in that the main focus is on a good, tight fit into the arch (because of the soft material being used). Another goal is the proper formation of relief areas that need less contact. The following steps are used to prepare the foot for making the orthotic:

1. Any area of callus, breakdown, or prominence needing relief should be covered with felt, foam, or some other material so that it will make a larger indentation on the heated orthotic material.

2. After this relief area is built up, the foot must be covered with a heavier protective covering than usual to avoid pain in sensitive areas as the hot material is put on. The authors use heavy socks, two pairs of socks, or double-thickness stockinette.

With regard to choosing a suitable material for the orthotic, Plastazote 1 or 2 is usually soft enough to feel comfortable under the most sensitive foot. Type of shoe is the major factor in choosing the thickness of material. For many women's shoes, the choice of thickness must be the thinnest possible (3/16-inch Plastazote).

Many patients wear shoes with high heel counters and ample toe box room. For these patients an extra-thick insole may be fashioned by gluing together two pieces of Plastazote and heating or by using a convection oven to autoadhere the two pieces together. The length of the pieces may be determined by pulling out the insole of the shoe to measure it or by using the length of the shoe as a guide.

When molding the material to a rheumatoid foot, we do not attempt to maintain subtalar neutral. Several authors agree on this point (Glass et al., 1982; Hertzman, 1973; Holmes, 1980; Jahss, 1991; McPoil & Brocato, 1985; Yale, 1987). A device that does not attempt to maintain the foot in the subtalar neutral position is called an accommodative orthotic.

The following steps are taken when making orthotics for the rheumatoid or a similar foot.

1. As detailed previously, the foot is prepared by padding any areas where relief is desired with extra felt or foam. A double-thickness of stockinette or sock protects the foot.

2. The patient is seated in a chair low enough so that the knee is at 90 degrees while maintaining the foot flat on the floor. A small foam pad is placed beside the foot.

3. One or two pieces of soft Plastazote (depending on desired thickness) are placed in a convection oven at 350 °F (175 °C).

When the material is malleable (or auto-adhered if a double-thickness), it is removed from the oven and placed on the foam (Figure 9.1).

4. The patient's foot is placed on the Plastazote with care being taken to center the foot so that the material shows 1 to 2 inches (25 to 50 mm) on all sides. The front needs to be at least the length of the insole (Figure 9.2).

5. As the patient puts progressively more weight onto the material, the clinician places one hand under the material and gently presses it up into the arch area. The patient may stand to add weight on the desired relief areas. Standing is not necessary if no relief areas are desired. The patient is cautioned not to place undue weight on the heel when standing unless a deep heel cup is desired (Figure 9.3).

6. The patient's foot is removed from the material.

7. The orthotic is trimmed with the shoe insole being used as a template if possible. If the insole is not removable, the bottom of the shoe may be used to estimate the length and width necessary (Figure 9.4).

8. As the device is trimmed, it should be placed into the shoe to check the fit. If the edges ride up inside the shoe, the device needs to be retrimmed. Remember that cutting material is just like cutting hair; it is easier to cut it off than to put it back on. The lesson here is to cut a little at a time and continually recheck the fit of the shoe (Figure 9.5).

9. When the device is nearly the correct size for the shoe, bevel the sides and rear so that they are perpendicular (or beyond). This angling allows a very snug fit in the shoe (Figure 9.6, a & b).

10. To extend the life of the orthotic, extra material may be added to the under surface. This added material may be in the form of an extra layer covering the entire bottom of the orthotic or an extra piece of material in the arch. Either of these may be added by use of contact cement. Remember to coat both surfaces to be glued together, and do not place the surfaces together until the contact cement has dried on both. The cement

loses its shiny look as it dries and takes on a dull finish (Figure 9.7).

11. Depending on the thickness of the material used, extra grinding may be possible to ensure a flat surface on the bottom of the orthotic (Figure 9.8).

12. Precautions outlined in chapter 11 are reviewed with the patient before the orthotics are used. Break-in time may need to be longer than normal, according to the amount of deformity or sensitivity of the foot.

Making an Orthotic for a Rheumatoid Foot

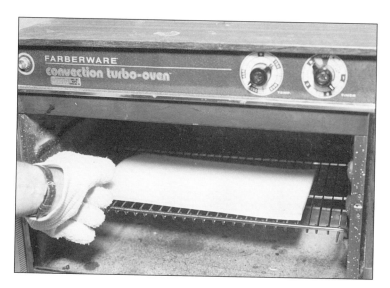

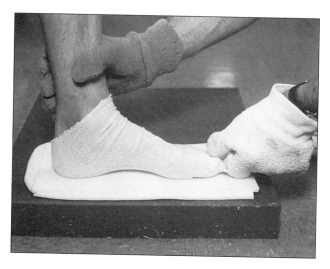

Figure 9.1 One or two layers of material, according to desired thickness, are placed in the oven.

Figure 9.2 Foot is placed on the material with a clear margin all around.

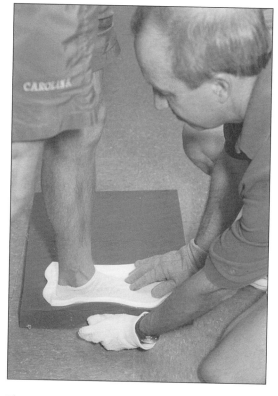

Figure 9.3 Support the arch as the patient applies weight.

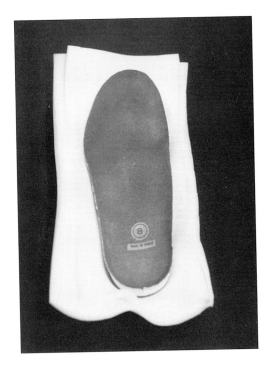

Figure 9.4 The shoe insole may be used as a template to size the orthotic.

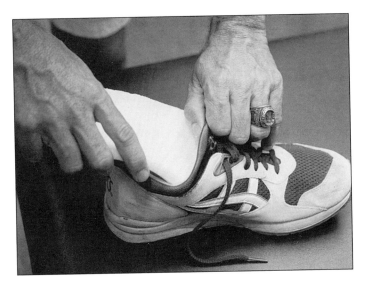

Figure 9.5 As cutting progresses, periodically place the orthotic into the shoe to check fit.

Figure 9.6 Bevel the sides (a) and rear (b) of the orthotic for proper fit.

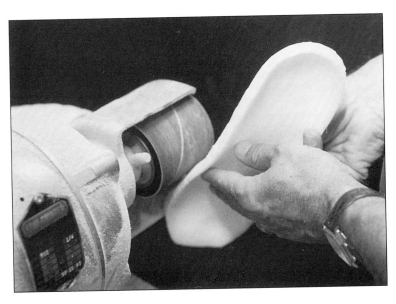

a

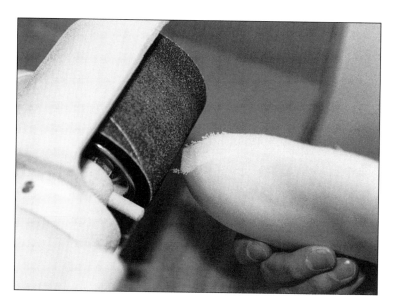

Figure 9.6b

Figure 9.7 Extra arch material may be glued in.

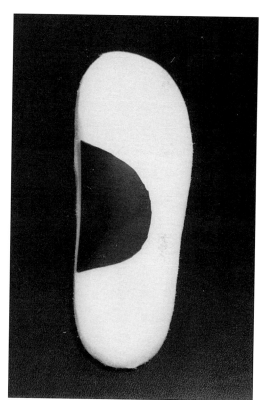

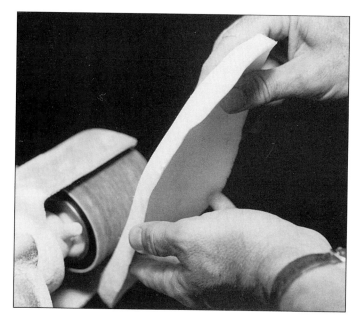

Figure 9.8 Some grinding of the bottom may be necessary to provide a flat surface.

Turf Toe

Turf toe is a common injury to the first metatarso-phalangeal joint of the foot. The mechanism of the injury is usually hyperextension of the meta-tarsophalangeal joint with the forefoot planted on the ground, as illustrated in Figure 9.9. The term *turf toe* is somewhat misleading in that the injury can occur on any type of terrain surface and in a variety of athletic activities. However, it is frequently seen in athletes who participate on synthetic surfaces. Rodeo, O'Brien, Warren, Barnes, Wickiewicz, and Dillingham (1990) report that 83 percent of the professional football players in their study sustained the injury on artificial turf. The combination of the rigidity of the surface and the flexibility of the shoe worn on synthetic surfaces contributes to the injury.

Orthotic Intervention

The initial goal in the management of turf toe is to stabilize and restrict the amount of dorsiflexion in the first metatarsophalangeal joint, which is accomplished by the orthotic. However, a comprehensive treatment plan incorporates other appropriate therapeutic modalities, exercise, rest, and protection from further trauma.

Because the forefoot is the area that needs support, the orthotic must be full length. The orthotic device is not posted since its purpose is to provide stability, not to correct biomechanical problems. Support can be provided in a variety of ways. A full-length orthotic or insole can be fabricated of a suitable semirigid to rigid material such as Orthoplast and placed in the shoe to limit extension (Figure 9.10). Visnick (1987) describes a method of Orthoplast fabrication combined with taping to restrict movement. Another option is to fabricate a semirigid device with rigid forefoot extension, as illustrated in Figure 9.11. A piece of rigid material can be placed between two thin layers of soft or semirigid material. A checkrein-type strap that wraps around the toe can be molded to the athlete's toe to prevent excessive extension.

Shoe Modification

Lack of rigidity in the forefoot portion of the shoe is a major contributor to turf toe. Many athletes wear turf shoes or basketball-type shoes while playing on synthetic surfaces. These types of shoes generally do not provide adequate forefoot rigidity to prevent excessive movement at the first metatarsophalangeal joint. Shoes with a steel shank that provide rigidity can be purchased. However, some athletes do not tolerate this type of athletic footwear well, so other means of adding support must be employed. A simple method of increasing the rigidity of the shoe is to insert a rigid insole. Orthoplast and similar materials are frequently used. An alternative is to insert a steel spring plate into the shoe. In addition to protecting the traumatized

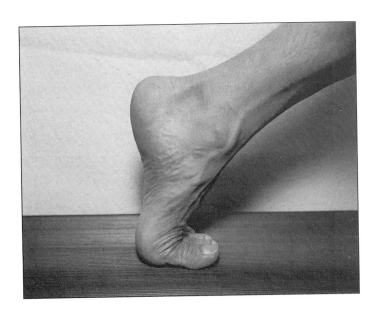

Figure 9.9 Mechanism of injury with turf toe, hyperdorsiflexion of the first metatarsophalangeal joint.

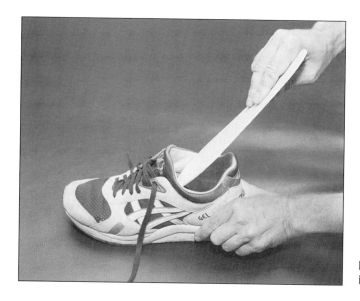

Figure 9.10 Full-length Orthoplast insole to stabilize turf toe.

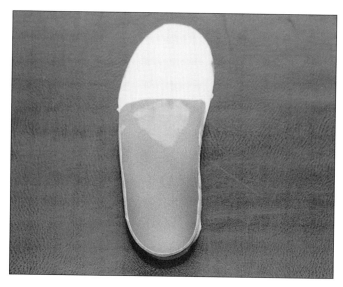

Figure 9.11 A semirigid orthotic with a rigid forefoot extension used in management of turf toe.

joint during the initial stages of the injury, active and passive range of motion is begun to maintain, and in some cases increase, the range of the joint to prevent reinjury.

Taping

Taping the toe to limit hyperextension can be an adjunct to shoe modification or orthotic intervention. The principle behind taping is to restrict the amount of extension in the joint. Several authors have described methods of taping the toe to limit dorsiflexion (Cibulka, 1990; Rodeo, O'Brien, Warren, Barnes, & Wickiewicz, 1989; Sammarco, 1988). Position the great toe in approximately 15 degrees of plantar flexion.

For maximal support, the tape is applied directly to the skin. The skin should be prepped with an appropriate tape adhesive. Place an anchor strip of 1.5-inch (40 mm) tape around the midfoot. Using 1-inch Elastikon tape (Johnson & Johnson), run strips of tape from the dorsal aspect of the foot to the plantar aspect of the foot, thereby pulling the toe in a plantar-flexed direction (Figure 9.12). An alternative technique is to cross the tape over the joint, as shown in Figure 9.13. Another method of adding stability is by the use of precut moleskin strips. The strip is fastened to the distal interphalangeal joint of the toe and secured to the midfoot with the toe in a plantar-flexed position (Figure 9.14).

Techniques for Limiting Toe Hyperextension

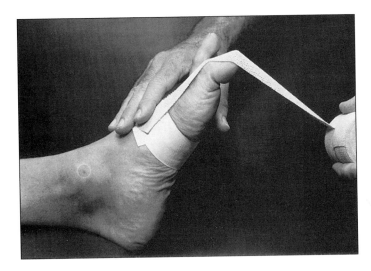

Figure 9.12 Turf toe taping. Note the direction of pull of the tape is from the dorsal aspect of the foot to the plantar aspect to limit dorsiflexion of the great toe.

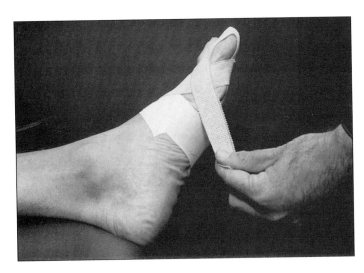

Figure 9.13 Alternative method for taping turf toe. Note that strips pull across the joint but still pull the toe in a plantar direction.

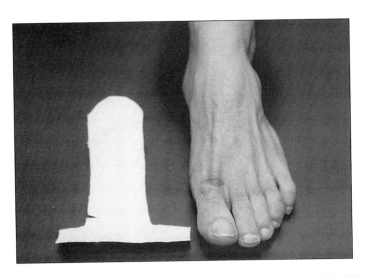

Figure 9.14 Precut strips of moleskin wrap around the toe to maintain a plantar flexed position.

Sesamoiditis

Sesamoiditis manifests as pain near the first metatarsophalangeal joint. Axe and Ray (1988) introduced the idea of a "J pad" to relieve pressure under the sesamoids (Figure 9.15). The pad can be fabricated out of orthopedic felt, PPT, or Spenco. The upper length of the J-shaped pad extends along the second metatarsal, with the curve of the J dipping proximal to the sesamoids. Pressure relief under a bony prominence is an easy and effective method of relieving symptoms in sensitive areas of the plantar aspect of the foot.

Metatarsalgia

Metatarsalgia, symptomized by pain in the forefoot, is one of the most commonly reported conditions in the foot (Cailliet, 1983). Since metatarsalgia is considered a catchall term, it is critical to have an accurate assessment of the foot before beginning treatment. The causes of metatarsalgia vary and can include vascular, avascular, neurogenic, or mechanical origins (Gould, 1989). Root, Orien, and Weed (1977)

state that abnormal pronation is the most common biomechanical problem that can cause metatarsalgia. McPoil and Schuit (1986) present a similar view in describing how a forefoot varus deformity can prolong the time the subtalar joint is pronating, causing the patient to push off on a hypermobile foot. This hypermobility can cause additional stresses at the forefoot. If biomechanical examination reveals any of these abnormal functions, then fabrication of an orthotic device is indicated.

The simplest method of relieving stress to the metatarsals is the use of a metatarsal pad. Holmes and Timmerman (1990) confirm that, when properly positioned, metatarsal pads are effective in reducing pressure to the metatarsal heads. A metatarsal pad can be applied directly to the patient or incorporated into an orthotic device. In either case, placement of the pad is critical. In order to relieve stress, the pad must be proximal to the metatarsal heads, as illustrated in Figure 9.16. Metatarsal pads can be cut from orthopedic felt or foam, or purchased prefabricated and cut to the proper size. Prefabricated orthotic shells can be purchased with a metatarsal pad incorporated into the device, as shown in Figure 9.17.

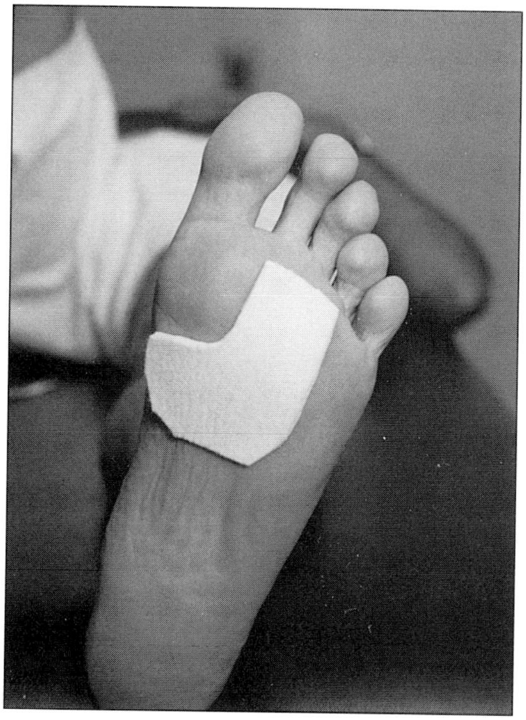

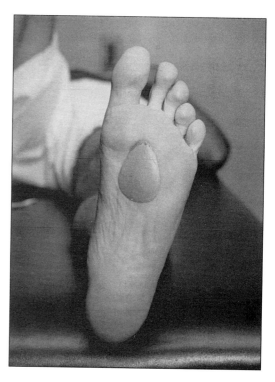

Figure 9.15   J pad relieves pressure on sesamoids.

Figure 9.16   Metatarsal pad placed proximal to the metatarsal head.

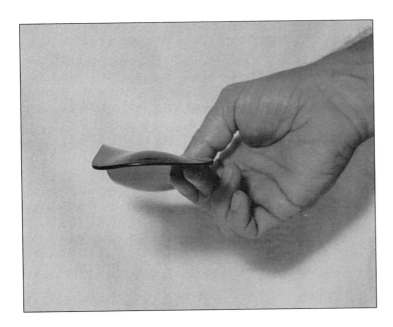

Figure 9.17 Orthotics can be purchased with metatarsal lifts incorporated into the shell.

When constructing a semirigid orthotic, a metatarsal pad can be placed between two layers of material while the material is being molded to the foot. Another technique is to make an intrinsic metatarsal lift, using your thumbs to create the lift just proximal to the painful metatarsal as the orthotic is molded to the patient, as illustrated in Figure 9.18 (Lutter, 1980). Another option is a metatarsal bar placed proximal to the metatarsal heads to relieve abnormal stress (Figure 9.19).

The use of orthopedic felt or similar materials is an inexpensive and effective method of reducing excessive pressure on the plantar aspect of the foot. As an added benefit, these types of materials can promote transfer of weightbearing stresses back to areas of the foot that are not bearing their share. The amount of stress or absence of weightbearing stress on the metatarsals can be classified into one of four categories (Doxey, 1985):

- First ray overload
- First ray insufficiency
- Central ray overload
- Central ray insufficiency

The rationale for treatment is to relieve the areas of overload by cutting out relief areas or by adding material to areas that are not bearing weight. Additional methods of orthotic modification for metatarsal and calcaneal pain are illustrated in Figures 9.20 and 9.21.

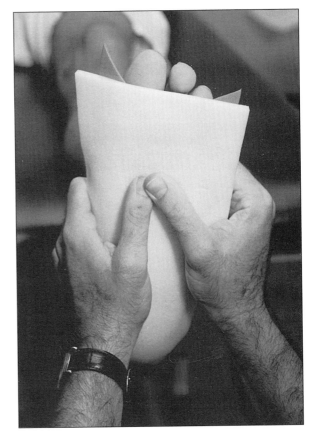

Figure 9.18 Use your thumbs to create an intrinsic metatarsal lift as the material is molded to the foot.

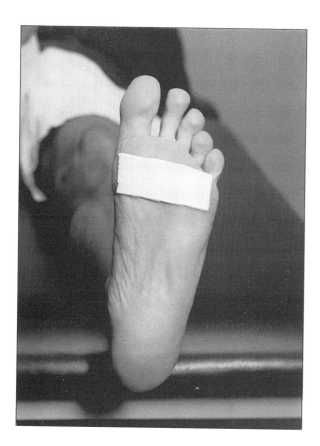

Figure 9.19 A metatarsal bar.

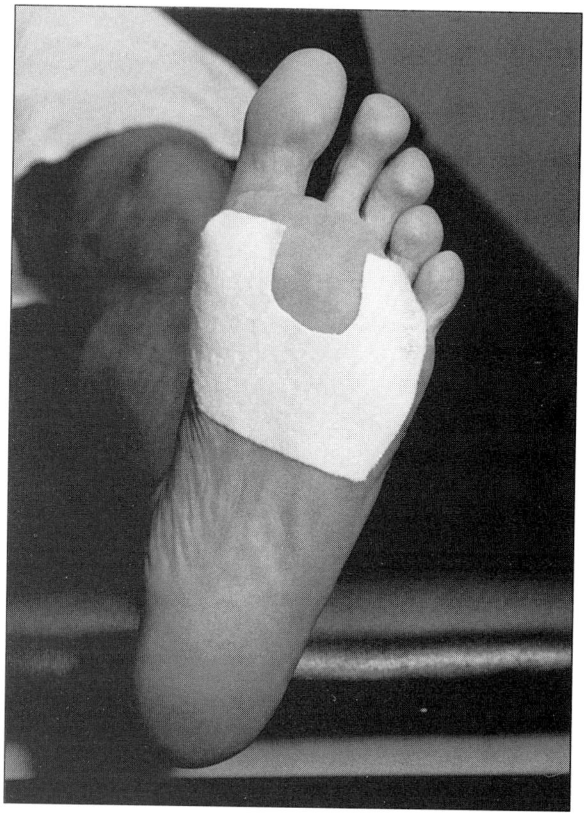

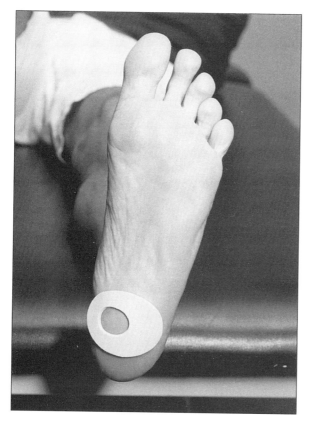

Figure 9.20 Cutting a relief area under the central metatarsals.

Figure 9.21 Relief area for a painful area of the heel.

Interdigital Neuromas

Interdigital neuromas are caused by entrapment of the interdigital nerve as it passes between the metatarsal heads. It is most commonly encountered between the third and fourth toes (Cailliet, 1983). Orthotic management of this condition would include the use of a metatarsal pad or bar. Mann (1984) recommends a metatarsal pad and a soft broad-toe shoe. If the neuroma is a result of pronation leading to forefoot hypermobility, a biomechanical orthotic would be indicated.

Plantar Fasciitis

Plantar fasciitis is an inflammation of the plantar fascia and the perifascial structures (Kwong, Kay, Voner, & White, 1988). Frequently seen in long distance runners, this condition usually responds to conservative treatment. The causes of plantar fasciitis are multiple and not fully understood. Kibler, Goldberg, and Chandler (1991) report isokinetic strength and flexibility deficits of the gastrocnemius and soleus complex as associated with plantar fasciitis. Their research re-emphasizes the need for assessing all factors that may be contributing to a pathological condition.

Orthotic devices can be a positive adjunct therapy for plantar fasciitis. If the biomechanical examination reveals abnormal pronation as a contributing factor, an orthotic device with appropriate modifications would be warranted.

Primary to the successful management of plantar fasciitis is control of the rearfoot movement. Kwong et al. (1988) recommend the use of a semirigid device that provides support for the first metatarsophalangeal joint, in addition to a shoe with a firm heel counter. Campbell and Inman (1974) report success with the University of California Biomechanical Laboratory (UCBL) device as a means of controlling pronation contributing to plantar fasciitis.

We have had success in cases of plantar fasciitis with fabrication of a deep heel cup that gives additional support. This heel cup is formed by molding heated Plastazote to the foot, as illustrated in Figure 9.22. The concept of heel cups is to stabilize the heel and increase shock absorption (Tanner & Harvey, 1988). Jørgensen (1990) concludes that a firm heel counter decreases muscle load at heel strike. The rubber-molded Tuli's brand heel cup is supportive and is perceived by wearers as the most comfortable of the commercially made devices.

Athletes that have plantar fasciitis should be encouraged to train in shoes that have a firm heel counter. Cutting out a relief area around the painful area may provide pain relief (Schepsis, Leach, & Gorzyca, 1991). An additional therapeutic tool is the use of the low-dye tape job. The objective of the tape job is to relieve stress on the plantar fascia. The effectiveness of the low-dye tape job is a good indicator of whether an orthotic device will be effective. Kosmahl and Kosmahl (1987) describe a method of low-dye taping with the foot in neutral subtalar joint position that we have found

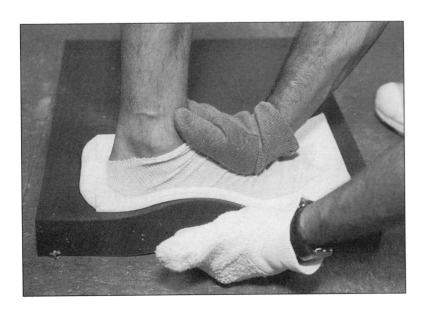

Figure 9.22 The athlete pushes down to create a deeper heel cup.

to be effective in reducing pain related to plantar fasciitis.

Many plantar fasciitis patients complain of initial pain after arising from bed in the morning. This results from the foot assuming a plantar-flexed and relaxed position during the night. Upon initial weightbearing, the plantar fascia is immediately stretched, causing pain. A recent adjunct therapy in the treatment of plantar fasciitis is the use of night splints (Figure 9.23). The purpose of the splint is to keep the ankle joint in a dorsiflexed position while the patient is sleeping. Wapner and Sharkey (1991) used the splints on 14 patients who were symptomatic for more than one year and achieved resolution of symptoms in 11 patients within 4 months.

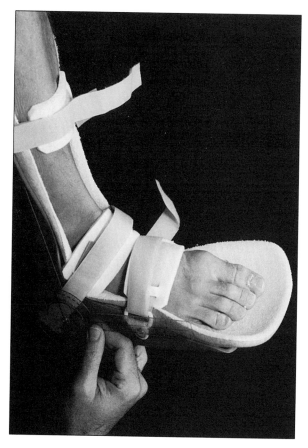

Figure 9.23 The use of a night splint is effective in the management of plantar fasciitis.

Summary

Orthotic devices may be adapted for special problems. These adaptations may include different materials, lengths, widths, depths, and areas of relief or prominence incorporated into the device. These changes to a regular orthotic, along with a comprehensive treatment plan, may successfully treat these unique orthopedic conditions.

References

Axe, M.J., & Ray, R.L. (1988). Orthotic treatment of sesamoid pain. *The American Journal of Sports Medicine*, **16**, 411–416.

Cailliet, R. (1983). *Foot and ankle pain* (2nd ed.). Philadelphia: Davis.

Campbell, J.W., & Inman, V.T. (1974). Treatment of plantar fasciitis and calcaneal spurs with the UC-BL shoe insert. *Clinical Orthopedics*, **103**, 57–62.

Cibulka, M.T. (1990). Management of a patient with forefoot pain: A case report. *Physical Therapy*, **70**, 41–55.

Coughlin, M. (1984). The rheumatoid foot. *Postgraduate Medicine*, **75**, 207–211.

Doxey, G.E. (1985). Management of metatarsalgia with foot orthotics. *The Journal of Orthopaedic and Sports Physical Therapy*, **6**, 324–333.

Glass, M., Karno, M., Sella, E., & Zeleznik, R. (1982). An office-based orthotic system in treatment of the arthritic foot. *Foot and Ankle*, **3**, 37–40.

Gould, J. (1982). Conservative management of the hypersensitive foot in rheumatoid arthritis. *Foot and Ankle*, **2**, 224–229.

Gould, J.S. (1989). Metatarsalgia. *Orthopedic Clinics of North America*, **20**, 553–562.

Hannaford, D. (1986). Soft orthoses for athletes. *Journal of the American Podiatric Medical Association*, **76**, 566–569.

Hertzman, C. (1973). Use of Plastazote in foot disabilities. *American Journal of Physical Medicine*, **52**, 289–303.

Holmes, D. (1980). Orthotics of the foot and ankle. In A. Helfet & D. Grubel-Lee (Eds.), *Disorders of the foot*. Philadelphia: Lippincott.

Holmes, G.B., & Timmerman, L. (1990). A quantitative assessment of the effect of metatarsal pads on plantar pressures. *Foot and Ankle*, **11**, 141–145.

Jahss, M.H. (1991). Arch supports, shielding, and orthodigita. In M. Jahss (Ed.), *Disorders of the foot and ankle* (pp. 2857–2866). Philadelphia: Saunders.

Jørgensen, U. (1990). Body load in heel-strike running: The effect of a firm heel counter. *The American Journal of Sports Medicine*, **18**, 177–181.

Kibler, W.B., Goldberg, C., & Chandler, T.J. (1991). Functional biomechanical deficits in running athletes with plantar fasciitis. *The American Journal of Sports Medicine*, **19**, 66–71.

Kosmahl, E.M., & Kosmahl, H.E. (1987). Painful plantar heel, plantar fasciitis, and calcaneal spur: Etiology and treatment. *The Journal of Orthopaedic and Sports Physical Therapy*, **9**, 17–24.

Kwong, P.L., Kay, D., Voner, R.T., & White, M.A. (1988). Plantar fasciitis mechanics and pathomechanics of treatment. *Clinics in Sports Medicine*, **7**, 119–126.

Lutter, L.D. (1980). Foot-related knee problems in the long distance runner. *Foot and Ankle*, **1**, 112–116.

Mann, R.A. (1984). Metatarsalgia: Common causes and conservative treatment. *Postgraduate Medicine*, **75**, 151–167.

McPoil, T.G., & Brocato, R.S. (1985). The foot and ankle: Biomechanical evaluation and treatment. In S. Gould & G. Davies (Eds.), *Orthopedic and sports physical therapy* (pp. 312–321). St. Louis: Mosby.

McPoil, T.G., & Schuit, D. (1986). Management of metatarsalgia secondary to biomechanical disorders. *Physical Therapy*, **66**, 970–972.

Mondl, A., Gardiner, J., & Bissett, J. (1969). The use of Plastazote in footwear for leprosy patients. *Leprosy Review*, **40**, 177–180.

Rodeo, S.A., O'Brien, S., Warren, R.F., Barnes, R., & Wickiewicz, T.L. (1989). Turf toe: Diagnosis and treatment. *The Physician and Sportsmedicine*, **17**, 132–147.

Rodeo, S.A., O'Brien, S., Warren, R.F., Barnes, R., Wickiewicz, T.L., & Dillingham, M.F. (1990). Turf-toe: An analysis of metatarsophalangeal joint sprains in professional football players. *The American Journal of Sports Medicine*, **18**, 280–285.

Root, M.L., Orien, W.P., & Weed, J.H. (1977). *Clinical biomechanics: Vol. II Normal and abnormal function of the foot*. Los Angeles: Clinical Biomechanics.

Sammarco, G.J. (1988). How I manage turf toe. *The Physician and Sportsmedicine*, **16**, 113–118.

Schepsis, A.A., Leach, R.E., & Gorzyca, J. (1991). Plantar fasciitis: Etiology, treatment, surgical results, and review of the literature. *Clinical Orthopaedics and Related Research*, **226**, 185–196.

Tanner, S.M., & Harvey, J.S. (1988). How we manage plantar fasciitis. *The Physician and Sportsmedicine*, **16**, 39–47.

Visnick, A.L. (1987). A playing orthosis of "turf toe." *Athletic Training*, **22**, 215.

Wapner, K.L., & Sharkey, P.F. (1991). The use of night splints for treatment of recalcitrant plantar fasciitis. *Foot and Ankle*, **12**, 135–138.

Yale, J.F. (1987). *Podiatric medicine*. Baltimore: Williams & Wilkins.

Orthotic Systems

10

Many practitioners feel that they do not have the time or expertise to build an orthotic from scratch. They prefer to use kits or systems with prefabricated pieces. In this chapter we will cover several products that encompass a wide range of orthotic fabrication capabilities.

Orthofeet

The Biothotic is an orthotic in kit form available from Orthofeet, Inc. of Hillsdale, New Jersey. It consists of a water-activated polymer sandwiched between a top cover and bottom shell of polyethylene foam. When water is added, the polymer expands, molds to the foot, and then sets within 3 minutes. The molding is done with the orthotic inside the shoe and the patient in weightbearing position. The Biothotic comes precut in full sizes only. There are four configurations of these orthotics:

- Profunction, a semirigid orthotic for excessive pronation or supination

- Sport Biothotic, a semirigid orthotic that incorporates an extra layer of foam for shock absorption

- Soft Biothotic, an orthotic that uses softer polyethylene foam and softer resin to provide cushion (designed for the hypersensitive foot, as in diabetic or rheumatoid conditions)

- High Heel, a model made very thin for dress shoes

Each pair of blanks costs approximately $30, except the Soft Biothotic and High Heel models,

which cost $35. The roller and needle injector come free with the first pair of orthotics purchased.

The following steps describe how to work with the Biothotic system:

1. Determine the type of orthotic to be used and the size. Since the sizes come only in full sizes, go to a size larger for half sizes requiring a full-length orthotic but to a size smaller for half sizes requiring a half-length orthotic. To check for correct size, the foot may be placed on the orthotic before it is removed from the pouch.

2. Remove the orthotic from its pouch. Place the orthotic into the shoe to ensure that it fits. Trim the cover extension for length and width. For three-quarter length orthotics, trim just proximal to the metatarsal heads. For half-length orthotics, trim 1/4 inch (6 mm) anterior to the edge of the bladder. These trims should follow a curve so that the extension under the medial side is slightly longer than on the lateral side. Care should be taken to avoid cutting into the bladder area so that the resin will not escape (Figure 10.1).

3. Bevel the edges with a grinder or pair of scissors so that the patient does not feel a drop-off at the anterior edge.

4. Have the patient try on the orthotic in the shoe.

5. Align the foot in neutral position. There are three ways: Tape the foot, place wedges on the orthotic, or place wedges on the bottom of the shoe. The wedges, which come prefabricated with adhesive on the back, are beveled to 3, 4, or 5 degrees. For shoes

with a lot of room, the company suggests posting the orthotic itself. For small shoes, the posts should be placed on the bottom of the shoe. For large deviations, posts on both the orthotic and outside of the shoe may be necessary to correct the problem. To post the rearfoot, always post on the bottom of the shoe to prevent interference with the resin (Figure 10.2).

6. Now that the foot is positioned in neutral, check to see that all the holes in the syringe are open by filling it from a cup of warm water and squirting the water out. If any holes are not open, use a pushpin to open them. Fill the syringe to the proper water level.

7. Turn the orthotic upside down; lift the vinyl cover from the medial injection hole and set it aside. Use your fingers to gently squeeze the medial arch area of the orthotic. Push the syringe into the hole, making sure it is all the way in and touching the bottom of the orthotic. Inject the water (Figure 10.3).

8. Shake the orthotic three or four times while the syringe is still in. Remove the syringe and put the tape cover back over the hole.

Use the roller provided or use your fingers to knead the injected area vigorously for 10 to 15 seconds (Figure 10.4).

9. Quickly insert the orthotic into the shoe and have the patient walk on it for 3 minutes. Check the orthotic for air bubbles. If one is found, puncture the area with a pushpin and knead to remove the air.

10. Replace the orthotic and have the patient walk for 2 more minutes. The temporary posts may be removed now also.

11. If the orthotic is correct, it should be worn for another 2 hours to ensure that the resin is set.

12. For permanent posting, the company suggests that the post be glued on with a super glue. For medial posting the company suggests two approaches: posting the rearfoot and forefoot separately, using the appropriately angled wedges, or posting a single wedge from the heel to a line 1/8 inch (3 mm) proximal to the metatarsal heads (Figure 10.5). For lateral posting the company suggests that the properly angled wedge be placed just distal to the heel, extending to a line 1/8 inch (3 mm) proximal to the metatarsal heads.

Using the Biothotic System

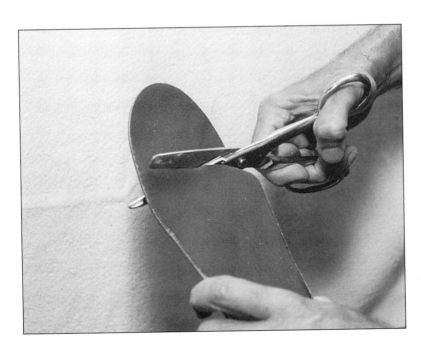

Figure 10.1 Trim 1/4 inch (6 mm) in front of the bladder, following a curved path so the medial side is slightly longer.

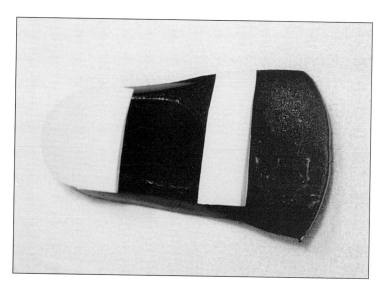

Figure 10.2 Company-supplied wedges may be applied to the orthotic as posting.

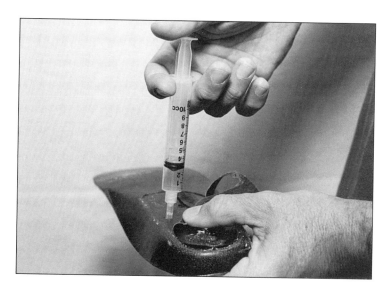

Figure 10.3 Inject room-temperature water.

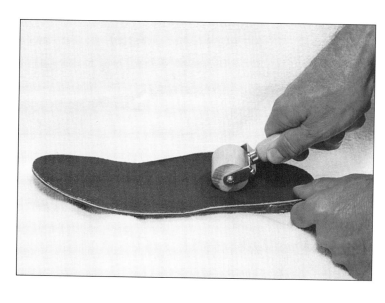

Figure 10.4 Roll or knead the injected area vigorously.

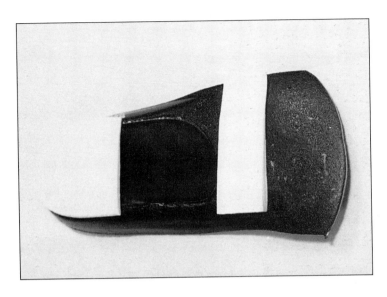

Figure 10.5 Permanent posting glued on medially.

Foot Technology

Foot Technology Inc. of St. Louis provides the components needed for the medical professional to fabricate a shock-absorbing, supportive, custom-molded orthotic quickly in the office. The system uses prefabricated thermoplastics for manufacture of orthotics in a manner similar to that described in chapter 7. The thermoplastic is molded directly to the patient's foot, posted, and ground during the same visit. The Foot Tech system consists of prefabricated insoles with a thermoplastic blank incorporated in between; a molding stand to position the foot in subtalar neutral when molding the insoles; half-sole supports that are glued to the insole, then ground and posted; a convection oven; and a grinder.

Technique

The procedure begins with the patient standing in the molding stand for a trial alignment (Figure 10.6). Subtalar neutral position is determined by palpation of the talar head and by visualization of the Achilles tendon. The knees should be slightly flexed with the support bar against the distal pole of the patella. Weight should be evenly distributed between the rearfoot and the forefoot.

The insole is heated at 250 °F (120 °C) for 2 to 3 minutes or until pliable. The insole is placed on the molding pillows and the foot positioned on the insole in subtalar neutral. The Foot Tech protocol describes molding both insoles simultaneously, but the authors have had better success molding them separately. After 2 minutes, the foot is removed from the insole. Additional arch support can be provided by placing the hand under the casting pillow during the insole molding (Figure 10.7). Half sole add-ons are glued to the insoles to provide additional control and support. With the appropriate density and size selected, the add-on is positioned on the insole. If necessary, the add-on can be heated until pliable to fit snugly against the insole. After the glue has dried, the insole and add-on are pressed together, and the edges are trimmed with scissors. The edges of the add-on are then ground, with care being taken not to damage the insole material. Finally the bottom of the add-on is ground to provide control and posting.

The Foot Tech system provides several types of insole materials and thicknesses along with add-ons of varying densities. This selection permits the fabrication of an orthotic that provides the patient the needed control and cushioning. The Foot Tech sales force describes their system as a "toolbox" for the manufacture of orthotics. It provides the tools needed to fabricate thermoplastic orthotics that are more durable and more smoothly finished than the Aliplast/Plastazote orthotics described in chapter 7.

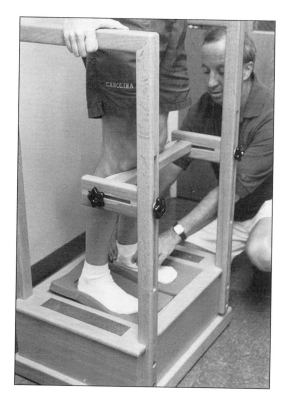

Figure 10.6 Patient on molding stand for trial alignment.

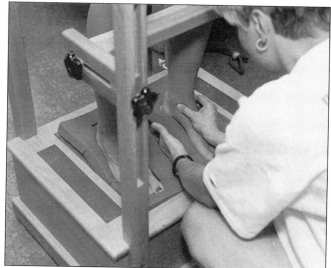

Figure 10.7 Placing hand under pillow provides additional support under the arch.

Amfit

Two of the latest high-tech inventions for foot orthotics are from Amfit, Inc. of San Jose, California: the Amfit Footfax Scanner and the Amfit Archcrafter milling system. Due to costs and complexity, this system is not for the occasional user. It is designed for the practitioner who does large numbers of orthotics daily. In fact some of the largest users of this equipment are the commercial orthotic manufacturers. As with many other improvements in existing technology, these devices are computer driven.

When using the Footfax Scanner (Figure 10.8), the patient's foot is positioned in subtalar neutral in weightbearing, semi-weightbearing, or non-weightbearing position over a contact scanner made of more than 500 posts (Figure 10.9). These posts mold to the contour of the foot and support the foot in this position. The scanner reads the deflection of each post and forms a digitized im-

age of the foot within the computer. This computer contour is recorded but may be modified by the operator. The operator can see the effect of any adjustment before it is entered as final data and manufacture of the orthotic begins. The software adjustments possible are:

- Inversion and eversion wedging up to 6 degrees
- Thickness control from 1 to 18 millimeters
- Arch support addition or subtraction from −30% to +30%.
- Sulcus rise from 1 to 9 millimeters
- Heel lifts from 1 to 9 millimeters

The Footfax Scanner information is stored in the computer or on floppy discs and may be pulled up later to make another set of orthotics or to adjust the present orthotic prescription. There also is an optional color printout, which shows the foot contour before and after the correction.

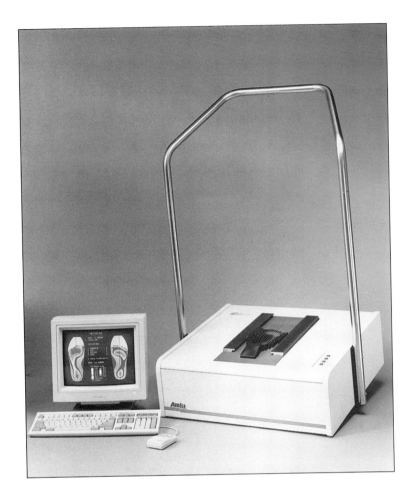

Figure 10.8   Footfax Scanner.

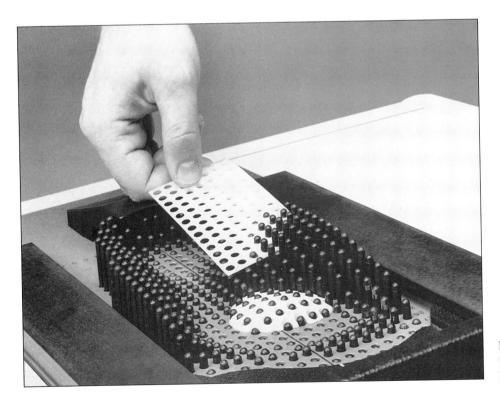

Figure 10.9   Scanner posts record foot position.

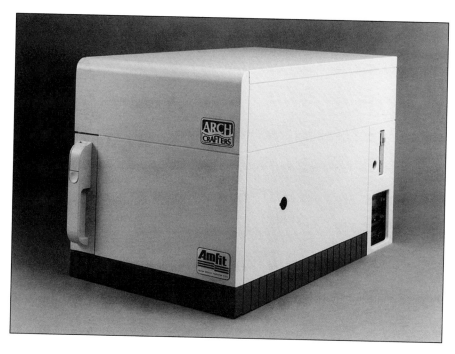

Figure 10.10 Archcrafter milling system.

The second component of the Amfit technology is the Archcrafter milling system (Figure 10.10). This part of the system may be on site with the scanner, or scanner information may be sent via modem to a central Archcrafter mill.

Before milling of the orthotic begins, the type of orthotic blank is selected from four available densities:

- Soft 43 to 48 C
- Medium 53 to 58 C
- Firm 73 to 80 C
- Dual-firm heel counter with medium field material

The milling device can produce up to four pairs of orthotics per hour.

Summary

There are a variety of orthotic systems or kits that aid in the fabrication of orthotics. These vary from simple orthotic kits to complex computer-assisted devices that actually fabricate the orthotic. The choice to use one of these systems is affected by the skill and expertise of the practitioner and by how much one wants to spend for an orthotic.

Practical Concerns of the Patient

11

Not all patients need an orthotic, and when prescribed the orthotic must be individualized for correct usage. The choice of orthotic has to match up appropriately with the patient's shoe type and training regimen, as well as with the diagnosed physical condition. In addition, the patient should understand the goals and limitations of orthotic therapy, using the orthotic properly, for treatment to be successful. In this chapter, we review issues that bear on individualizing orthotic treatment, including questions that patients commonly ask—or fail to ask.

Opinion varies as to the limitations of orthotic therapy. For example, Peter Cavanagh, professor of biomechanics at Penn State University, quoted by Murphy (1986), would rule out orthotics for competitive athletes altogether, contending that "competitive athletes should not have something loose such as orthotics or something which adds weight such as an orthotic. Orthoses have proven to be an effective device for correcting some of the malalignment problems in the recreational athlete."

Subotnick (1983) cautions that orthotics are overprescribed, poorly understood, and usually not integrated into an overall treatment plan. He identifies five problems that may be caused by orthotics:

- Excessive varum may cause iliotibial band syndrome.

- Neutral foot control may cause hip rotator strain.

- Excessive varum control may lead to trochanteric bursitis.

- Neutral foot control may lead to low back pain.

- Nonsoft devices may contribute to plantar fasciitis due to pressure in the plantar fascia at midstance or toe-off.

A failure rate as high as 15 percent is common in the treatment of runners' injuries according to Subotnick (1975), who offers six rules by which to make orthotics:

- Orthotics should be made from a neutral mold in most cases. Orthotic fabrication should be guided by the idea that erring toward an arch that is too little is better than erring toward an arch that is too high.

- Patients with tight posterior muscles of the leg require a non-neutral orthotic that is slightly pronated.

- The rearfoot post should control the foot at heel strike, but too much rearfoot post will not allow normal pronation to take place, putting abnormal stress on ankles and knees. A correct rearfoot post must allow 4 to 6 degrees of pronation to take place at heel strike.

- Patients must allow for break-in and should return for adjustments to the orthotic.

- Rigid orthoses work for activities such as distance jogging and are better suited for street shoes. Softer, semirigid orthoses are better suited for speed work, competition, and field events. Subotnick recommends that patients have two pairs of orthotics, one pair of each type.

- Not all problems need an orthotic as treatment.

Lutter (1981) gives four basic treatment tenets for any runner with a cavus foot experiencing pain or other symptoms: reduction of activity, pain management using modalities and medicine, additional stretching and strengthening, and orthotics.

Jahss (1991) uses the following principles for soft orthotics:

- Fixed deformities should never be corrected by raising the area under a callused area.
- The floor should be brought up to the foot in noncontact areas.
- Areas of excess pressure should have relief built in.
- Calluses are a good indication of too much pressure on an area.
- Areas that usually have little or no weight-bearing capabilities should have contact built into them. Good examples of these types of areas are the arch and distal arch just behind the metatarsal heads.

The Orthotic Appointment

Individualizing the orthotic to the patient formally begins on the day of the clinical appointment, but the process can be facilitated by a little preparation in advance. The patient should be advised beforehand to bring any shoes in which the orthotics may be used. The patient will try out the orthotic in all these shoes before leaving the clinic. Any orthotic devices that have been used in the past should be brought in also. The patient should be encouraged to wear shorts or some type of clothing conducive to biomechanical examination of the lower extremity.

Most orthotics will require that the shoe's insole be removed due to space limitations. This is to prevent the foot from coming out of the rear of the shoe or sliding due to the height of the rearfoot post. When solid semirigid orthotics are used, the rubber arch support of the shoe must be removed to prevent the arch of the orthotic being pushed too high. When rigid orthotics are used, the arch of the orthotic may clear the shoe arch cookie so that it may not need to be removed.

Removing the insole may be as simple as reaching into the bottom of the shoe and pulling out the insole, if the insole is not glued down. In other shoes, gentle force may be needed to separate the glued portion of the insole from the bottom of the shoe. Care should be taken to avoid leaving pieces of the foam from the insole stuck to the bottom of the shoe.

Break-In

Orthotics require a gradual getting used to, or accommodation. Even with a gradual regimen, some individuals never accommodate to them. In a study of 143 military recruits given foot orthotics, 21 percent had to discontinue use within 14 days due to discomfort (Milgrom et al., 1985). In a study of 109 patients receiving hard orthotics, 40 percent experienced problems in the fit. Most common (40 percent) were problems in the arch area; heel slippage (31 percent) was the next most common problem (Blake and Denton, 1985).

Just like new shoes, an orthotic device requires a break-in period. Patients must adapt to the new relationship their feet have with the ground. This new relationship can adversely affect the entire lower extremity if the patient does not understand the need to allow a gradual accommodation. The length of time required to accommodate to an orthotic device varies according to the type of orthotic and the amount of deviation that is being treated. Each of the types of orthotics has its own characteristics that affect patient tolerance. Although hard orthotics do provide some flexibility and give, semirigid and soft devices require much less time for accommodation by the patient.

Philips (1990) offers the following suggestions for break-in of orthotics used in sports:

1. Wear the orthotic for 1 hour on the day of issue.
2. Increase the time for wearing the orthotic by 1 hour daily.
3. Once the orthotic has been worn all day, then sports may be started in the orthotic.
4. At first the orthotic should be worn for one-quarter of the time of the sporting event.
5. Increase the time for sports activity with the orthotic by one-quarter every 3 days.

McPoil and Brocato (1985) suggest that the patient wear the orthotics 2 hours the first day and increase this time by 1 hour daily. They allow sporting activities to begin after the orthotics have been worn by the athlete at least 6 to 8 hours daily.

The authors' instructions for a patient are as follows:

1. Wear the orthotic for 2 hours the first day.
2. Increase this time by 2 to 3 hours daily unless symptoms increase or new symptoms appear.
3. Once the orthotic has been worn all day, then sports use may begin.
4. During the first 2 days of sports use, the orthotic should be worn only one-third of the time. For example, if running 3 miles, the athlete would carry the orthotic in hand for 2 miles, then stop to insert the orthotic and finish the run.
5. Stop using the orthotic and phone us if symptoms increase or new problems arise. Blisters, calluses, or other unusual problems unrelated to the original problem are signs that the orthotic is not right or that the patient is making a mistake in the wear-in period. Cracchiolo (1982) believes that calluses are the most reliable sign of too much pressure.

Patient Expectations

One of the main points that needs to be explained to the patient is that orthotics do not provide overnight relief in a majority of cases. Problems that generate inflammation will not be alleviated quickly, short of anesthetic injection. Orthotics function by correcting the discrepancies that cause inflammation—not a quick process. Patients should not hastily judge the effectiveness of the orthotic. Our recommendation is that the patient wait at least 6 weeks before deciding on the benefits of the orthotic. If at the end of these 6 weeks the patient has seen no improvement in symptoms, then it is time to return to the clinic for reevaluation. This reevaluation covers not only the biomechanical aspects of the device but also patient compliance, knowledge of previous instructions, and wearing habits. More than once the authors have had patients return to clinic with severe complaints that were alleviated by switching the orthotics back to the proper left and right shoes.

Nesbitt (1992) encourages patients to report problems after they have worn the orthotic for about a week. He reports that 10 to 20 percent of patients need to have the orthotic adjusted on the first follow up visit. Hannaford (1986) suggests a break-in period of 30 to 50 miles for runners with semirigid orthoses. After this time, adjustments for fit and other corrections may be made.

The patient should be made to understand during the initial appointment that there are problems that do not respond to orthotic therapy. Other treatment methods may be used in conjunction with, or instead of, orthotic prescription, including exercises for strength or stretching, modalities, or, ultimately, surgery. Even when orthotics are indicated, the patient must comply with training instructions to reduce overuse problems. No device or therapy will be effective if the overuse is continued.

Longevity

Feet, like all other parts of anatomy, change with time. Patients are encouraged to have their orthotics checked every 2 to 4 years to ensure that the prescription should remain the same. In younger patients who are still growing, this recheck may need to be performed at least every year. Very seldom do we prescribe hard orthotics for young patients since the cost of replacement to keep up with growth would be prohibitive. Subotnick (1981) also suggests soft orthoses for growing children since soft orthotics can be replaced more frequently for less cost.

Semirigid orthotics made of heat moldable plastics wear out eventually due to compression or "bottoming out" of the material. The life expectancy of the material depends on usage and body weight. Seldom will they last over 1 or 2 years, even with moderate usage. Soft orthotics made of materials such as Plastazote will last an even shorter span. This material bottoms out rapidly and should be rechecked every 6 months. The recheck is especially critical for patients with diabetes or rheumatoid arthritis.

Patient Questions

Patients are encouraged to ask questions during the entire process. Below are listed some of the more frequently asked questions and answers.

1. *When should I expect my pain to go away?* Patients should be cautioned that orthotics are not a panacea. They are often used as a portion of the

overall treatment of a problem. Strict adherence to the entire treatment protocol is needed to enhance the effectiveness of the orthotics. This protocol may include additional exercises, drugs, or modalities. For most problems, the patient should note some improvement within 6 weeks. We tell patients to expect a gradual improvement, but if none is noted, schedule an appointment so that their program may be reviewed.

2. *Can I wear the orthotics in all shoes?* Many fashionable women's shoes will not accommodate regular orthotics due to space requirements. Several of the orthotic manufacturers sell a thinner, cut-down version of a hard orthotic that will fit in almost any shoe.

3. *What kind of shoe should I buy to use the orthotic in?* Orthotics take up space in a shoe. An extra-depth shoe or even a half-size increase may be necessary to accommodate both the foot and the orthotic (Cracchiolo, 1982; Jahss, 1991). Shoes with a removable insole are also a great help, allowing better fit and also giving a more even surface or foundation for the orthotic to sit on. Many orthotics are only as good as the shoes they are mounted in. For most pronators we suggest a moderately rigid shoe with good antipronation devices built in, such as dual-density midsoles, straighter last, boarded or combination last, or an external heel counter.

4. *How long will the orthotics last?* The answer depends on many variables. Depending on the weight and activities of the individual, semirigid orthotics made of heat-moldable plastics will last up to 2 years. Rigid orthotics made of materials such as Rohadur will last much longer. Some patients claim to have used the same hard orthotic for 10 or 12 years without the orthotic cracking. Due to changes in anatomy (such as weight loss and gain), foot structure, and flexibility, we feel that orthotics should be reevaluated every 2 to 4 years. The need for reevaluation is especially important if the patient's activity level increases.

5. *How will I know if I am having problems?* Symptoms such as blisters, calluses, and open wounds are late signs that something is amiss. Initially, the foot may have a slight red mark where pressure is too great. Any increase in symptoms of the original problem or new problems should be a warning that some aspect of the patient's program is not correct.

6. *How much will the orthotic cost?* Many factors influence cost. Having a greater number of people involved in the process tends to push the cost higher. Therefore, in-house fabrication is usually cheaper than sending out the molds. Commercial fabrication from a mold that is mailed to the company is often the most expensive option. Depending on the type of orthotic ordered, costs range from $60 to $350. Soft and semirigid orthotics usually cost in the $60 to $150 range. Hard orthotics made of TL-61 may cost as much as $350.

Problems and Solutions

Table 11.1 lists the most common problems patients have following orthotic application. Listed with these problems are the most common causes and solutions.

Advice to Runners

Because of the large number of runners seen in our clinics for orthotic evaluation, we have compiled a list of rules that we give runners as an adjunct to any therapy.

1. *Reduce mileage on hills.* Most runners know that running up a grade is hard on the extremities. Few runners realize that downhill running may be just as detrimental or even worse than uphill running. In some parts of the country, finding a level place to run may be extremely difficult. We suggest that a local track may be the only place that is level.

2. *Serious runners who train regularly should reverse their route every other day.* Many runners leave their door and make a sweeping right-hand turn and continue on a route of right turns until they circle back to the starting point. This pattern constantly puts extra strain on the outside leg to supinate and the inside leg to pronate (Sallade & Koch, 1992). To lessen this effect, the athlete should run the opposite routes every other day. Runners who run on a track also need to reverse their routes. For some reason, all the tracks in the world are meant to be run counterclockwise, which means that the pressure experienced by the outside leg in turns is being continually applied to the right leg. When a runner runs the opposite

Table 11.1   Causes and Solutions of Common Problems with Orthotics

Problem	Cause	Solution
Symptoms increase	Cast or posting incorrect	Reevaluate and recast
New injury	Overcorrection or wrong post	Reevaluate and re-do orthotic
Arch pain or blisters	Arch too high	Lower arch
	Top edge of orthotic not beveled well	Regrind
	Flexible cavus foot	Use soft material under arch
Painful metatarsal heads	Orthotic too long	Shorten orthotic
	Distal edge not beveled enough	Regrind
	Incorrect forefoot post	Reevaluate and repost
	Orthotic not broken in	Slow down break-in period
First metatarsal pain	Hallux rigidus	Add forefoot extension
	Plantar-flexed first ray	First metatarsal relief cut-out
Fifth metatarsal pain	Valgus post is too high	Decrease post
	Orthotic too high on lateral side	Shorten lateral edge
Blisters or cuts just proximal to metatarsal heads	Orthotic too short	Add extension or re-do
	Forefoot edge too high	Regrind forefoot post
Heel comes out of shoe	Orthotic too narrow	Full top insole or re-do device
	Shell material too slick	Roughen bottom of device with grinder, or double fold adhesive tape and place on bottom of device
Slipping off lateral side	High arch	Reevaluate and re-do
	Medial post is too high	Grind down medial post
	Abducted forefoot	Add lateral flange
	Slick material	Add top cover
Sesamoid pain increases or continues	Not enough rearfoot control	Increase rearfoot post, or use more rigid material
Lack of shock absorption symptoms occur	Overcorrection on posts	Reduce post angles
	Overcontrol	Reevaluate/use softer material
Knee pain or shin pain continues	Not enough control	Reevaluate
		Use more rigid material, or increase post
Bunion pain	Orthotic exceeds proper height	Reduce post
		Remove shoe insert
		Re-do orthotic with thinner material

way around a track, it is important to be aware of the danger of collisions. The outside lane may be the best course on days when clockwise running is performed.

Runners who run on crowned or sloping surfaces may also overstress one leg (Figure 11.1).

The runner who always runs facing traffic on a crowned road will oversupinate on the downhill leg and overpronate on the uphill leg (Sallade & Koch, 1992). To correct this bias, the runner should avoid crowned surfaces or at least alternate the downhill and uphill legs when possible.

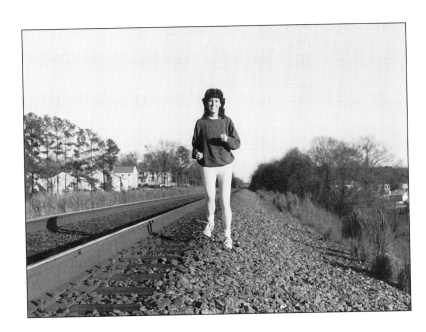

Figure 11.1 Running on a crowned or sloping surface may cause a leg length problem.

3. *Avoid sudden changes in surfaces.* Much has been written about the disadvantages of running on hard surfaces. Subotnick (1981) writes that running on a hard, unyielding surface can lead to injury. He states that the flat foot has too much mobility and the high-arched foot has too little mobility for hard surfaces. In our experience, the problems begin not from running on a hard or soft surface but from being accustomed to running on one type of surface and suddenly changing to another surface. This problem is particularly evident when runners go from a surface such as asphalt to a surface such as sand at the beach.

4. *Increase mileage very slowly.* The body is a great adapter to stress, as long as the stress is added gradually. A study by James, Bates, and Osternig (1978) of 180 running patients showed that 60 percent of injuries were due to training errors, with 29 percent of these due to excessive mileage. Lysholm and Wiklander (1987) found that 60 percent of the patients in their study had injuries caused by extrinsic factors such as excessive mileage or sudden increases in training routine. In a review of three epidemiological studies on running, Powell, Kohl, Caspersen, and Blair (1986) showed that in all three studies mileage was the factor most closely associated with running injuries. A particularly troublesome habit, especially among college students, is the failure to reduce mileage after taking a break from running during a holiday. After a layoff, mileage should be reduced so that the body has a chance to readjust.

5. *Replace shoes frequently, but don't change shoe types or brands unless a problem occurs.* Most midsoles of shoes will bottom out around 500 to 600 miles (Figure 11.2). Runners should keep track of their mileage and replace shoes as they near this mileage. Mileage must be the key to replacement since the appearance of the shoe will not show the bottoming effect. Runners should not change brands or types of shoes if they are not having problems. In other words, "Don't get off a winning horse." If a runner finds a model of a shoe that is functioning well, it is a good idea to buy many pairs at one time. The shoe companies have a bad habit of stopping production of a model after a short time for no apparent reason.

6. *Don't expect overnight miracles from stretching.* The first thing many runners question when an injury occurs is their stretching habits. Stretching is always an important part of our treatment regimen but almost never the entire treatment. Many runners feel that increased stretching will counteract any training error or overuse problem. This simply is not true. We encourage runners to stretch but with realistic expectations. Stretching, like strengthening, needs to be performed routinely for months before the benefits are realized. We instruct our runners to stretch gently before they run and to warm up gradually. The bulk of stretching may be done after the run to take advantage of warm muscles. Stretching during cooldown has been reported to decrease next-day muscle soreness.

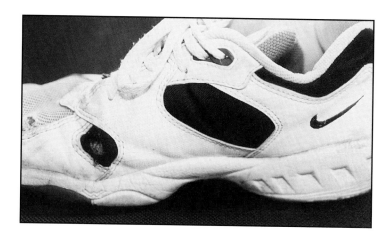

Figure 11.2 A shoe with a bottomed out midsole.

Summary

The type and configuration of orthotics is a source of controversy. The ideas concerning fabrication of orthotics by several authors have been presented. Once the orthotic is fabricated, a proper break-in will be required. The patient should be encouraged to ask questions about the use of orthotics and should be encouraged to return to the clinic should problems occur. Many of these problems may be addressed through reevaluation and modification of the orthotic. Many injuries are the result of training errors. Simple tips to prevent these training errors have been offered in this chapter and should eliminate many injuries caused by overuse or errant training.

References

Cracchiolo, A. (1982). Office treatment of adult foot problems. *Orthopedic Clinics of North America, 13*, 515.

Hannaford, D. (1986). Soft orthoses for athletes. *Journal of the American Podiatric Medical Association, 76*, 566–569.

Jahss, M. (1991). Arch supports, shielding and orthodigita. In M. Jahss (Ed.), *Disorders of the foot and ankle* (pp. 2857–2866). Philadelphia: Saunders.

James, S., Bates, B., & Osternig, L. (1978). Injuries to runners. *American Journal of Sports Medicine, 6*, 40–50.

Lutter, L. (1981). Cavus foot in runners. *Foot and Ankle, 1*, 225–228.

Lysholm, J., & Wiklander, J. (1987). Injuries in runners. *The American Journal of Sports Medicine, 15*, 168–170.

McPoil, T., & Brocato, R. (1985). The foot and ankle: Biomechanical evaluation and treatment. In J. Gould & G. Davies (Eds.), *Orthopedic and sports physical therapy* (pp. 300–341). St. Louis: Mosby.

Milgrom, C., Giladi, M., Kashtan, H., Simkin, A., Chisin, R., Marguiles, J., Steinberg, R., Aharson, Z., & Stein, M. (1985). A prospective study on the effect of a shock absorbing orthotic device on the incidence of stress fractures in military recruits. *Foot and Ankle, 6*, 101–103.

Murphy, P. (1986). Orthoses: Not the sole solution for running ailments. *The Physician and Sportsmedicine, 14*, 164–167.

Nesbitt, L. (1992). A practical guide to prescribing orthoses. *The Physician and Sportsmedicine, 20*, 76–87.

Philips, J. (1990). *The functional foot orthosis.* New York: Churchill Livingstone.

Powell, K., Kohl, H., Caspersen, C., & Blair, S. (1986). An epidemiological perspective on the causes of running injuries. *The Physician and Sportsmedicine, 14*, 100–114.

Sallade, J., & Koch, S. (1992). Training errors in long distance running. *Athletic Training, 27*, 50–53.

Subotnick, S. (1975). The abuses of orthotic devices. *Journal of the American Podiatry Association, 65*, 1025–1027.

Subotnick, S. (1981). The flat foot. *The Physician and Sportsmedicine, 9*, 85–91.

Subotnick, S. (1983). Foot orthoses: An update. *The Physician and Sportsmedicine, 11*, 103–109.

Index

About the Authors

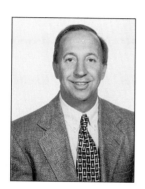

Skip Hunter, PT, ATC, is director of sports medicine for the Clemson Sports Medicine and Rehabilitation Center in Clemson, South Carolina. Before joining the Clemson center, he was director of sports medicine at The Charlotte Sports Center. In addition, Hunter spent eight years as a football trainer for the University of North Carolina at Chapel Hill—three years as an assistant and five years as head trainer. In 1989 and 1991, he also served as trainer for the United States Soccer Program.

Hunter teaches continuing education courses throughout the country and has had articles published in a variety of publications including *The National Athletic Trainers Journal, The Physician and Sportsmedicine, The Journal of Orthopedics and Sports Physical Therapy*, and *The Journal of the American Physical Therapy Association.*

Hunter is a member of the National Athletic Trainers Association (NATA) and the sports medicine section of the American Physical Therapy Association (APTA).

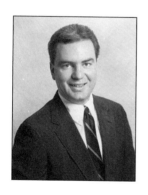

Michael G. Dolan, MA, ATC, CSCS, is an associate professor of sports medicine and exercise sciences at Canisius College in Buffalo, New York. He has taught both the theory and the practice of orthotic fabrication to hundreds of students and clinicians, and has been making his own orthotics for 12 years. In addition to his work in foot orthotics, Dolan conducts research on edema control at the University of Buffalo.

Dolan is a column editor for the journal *Athletic Therapy Today.* He has written several abstracts for the National Reviewer for the association's journal. He also serves on NATA's evaluation team for program accreditation and belongs to NATA's New York State chapter, where he acts as chair of the scholarship committee.

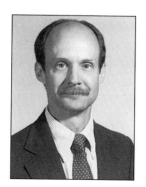

John M. Davis, PT, ATC, is a licensed physical therapist and athletic trainer at the University of North Carolina at Chapel Hill (UNC), where he has worked for the Division of Sports Medicine since 1975. He has served as athletic trainer and physical therapist for the UNC men's basketball team since 1977.

Davis is a contributing author to *Therapeutic Modalities in Sports Medicine* and *Rehabilitation Techniques in Sports Medicine*, both edited by William Prentice. He has also published articles in the *National Athletic Trainers Journal* and the *Journal of Orthopedics and Sports Physical Therapy.* Davis is a member of the NATA and the sports medicine section of the APTA.

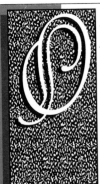

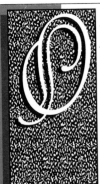ther titles from *Human Kinetics*

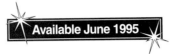
The definitive how and why of athletic taping and bracing

Athletic Taping and Bracing

David H. Perrin, PhD, ATC
1995 • Cloth • Approx 136 pp • Item BPER0502
ISBN 0-87322-502-3 • Call for price.

Strategies for passing the NATA certification exam

Lorin Cartwright, MS, EMT, ATC
1995 • Paper • 264 pp • Item BCAR0504
ISBN 0-87322-504-X • $25.00 ($33.50 Canadian)

Preparing
for the
Athletic
Trainers'
Certification
Examination

LORIN CARTWRIGHT

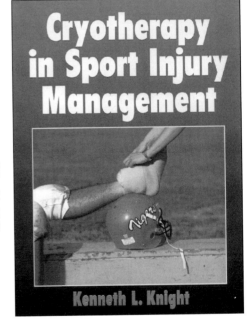

Cryotherapy in Sport Injury Management

Kenneth L. Knight

Cold therapy comprehensively explained

Kenneth L. Knight, PhD, ATC
1995 • Paper • 312 pp • Item BKNI0771
ISBN 0-87322-771-9 • $26.00 ($36.50 Canadian)

Prices subject to change.

**Human
Kinetics**

2335

To place order: U.S. customers call **TOLL FREE 1 800 747-4457**;
customers outside of U.S. use the appropriate telephone number/address
in the front of this book.

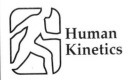